THE MOST
Unforgettable
ER NIGHT SHIFT EVER

C. ADAMS

ISBN 978-1-66789-328-0 ebook 978-1-66789-329-7

Contents

Preface

After twenty-five years working as an emergency physician, I have experienced a lot. At times, I have felt like I was riding a roller coaster without a safety bar. By reading this book, I am offering you a memorable seat without having to risk life or limb. I must warn you that there will be moments when you may feel your stomach stuck in your throat. After hair-raising descents, be prepared for some twists and turns. I promise a unique ride that will be memorable while avoiding heartbreaking and lethal encounters. For you, those encounters will sometimes be humorous, and thankfully, everybody lives. This medical story is sometimes less eloquent and more off color than you have probably read before. The ER cases presented will veer from the usual tragic to the more titillating. If a case happens to be sad, I'll only present the ones that I feel are sensational. Entertainment in the form of humor is what I have decided to embrace. So instead of fatal cases, you will see funny and absurd cases. But real!

I hate to admit it, but after my first two decades in the trenches, I needed more motivation. My career goal of earning money by helping people wasn't enough. As a result, I developed my three E's of emergency medicine: entertainment, education, and enlightenment. I believe life should include entertainment as well as excitement. If work can provide that, one can consider themself lucky. In addition, learning should be a goal as we travel this existence. One stagnates in life without growing in knowledge. Lastly, I equate enlightenment with being struck by a life-affirming or possibly a game-changing event. Focusing on those three areas has allowed me to once again be recharged and enjoy the ride. It is why I decided to follow the three E's while writing this book. First, this book should be entertaining. I selected personal cases that were unforgettable. Along the way, I have added medical insight to provide you with some education. Learning is much easier if you are having fun while being informed. My hope is that you will gain some insight while reading about individuals who were experiencing health care emergencies. Gleaning gems of wisdom from other people's mistakes is an easy way to obtain intelligence without receiving your own scars.

The chronicle that follows is difficult to classify. I endeavored to write a nonfiction account of some of my most bawdy patient encounters. By far, the majority of the depictions and descriptions are facts. However, in order to make the cases interconnected and protect the anonymity of those involved, I had to change some details. Still, this work could be most accurately described as an autobiography with an added information manual for the ER. Every one of the cases presented truly existed. Also, in all but one case, every patient was actually one of my patients. The one deviation was a case that my senior chief emergency resident experienced. That encounter was not only racy but dealt with a life-threatening situation that relied on a physician's full investigative armamentarium, thus making it a great learning case. This book will take you through a single twelve-hour night shift. As the night shift progresses, I assist with defining medical jargon and include further educational insight that would benefit anyone who may someday be an ER patient. Hopefully, after you complete the ride, you will learn what my emergency health care team does on an extreme Saturday night. Maybe you'll gain enough insight to avoid being a patient yourself. Enjoy!

Introduction

Finishing my supper of leftover spaghetti and meatballs, I place a peanut butter and jelly sandwich, three chocolate chip cookies, and some salty snacks into my lunch bag. Fuel in one hand, I grab my stethoscope with the other as I head out the door to get into my truck. I am wearing a white T-shirt and my blue scrub bottoms. I will put my matching blue scrub top over my T-shirt when I reach the hospital parking lot. The sun still had a couple hours before setting, but most of my twelve-hour shift would be during complete darkness. However, that evening had something special about it. Truthfully, most health care workers, especially those who work in the Emergency Department (ED), wouldn't use the word "special," but would more likely prefer the term "ominous" to describe their feelings about the upcoming evening. Tonight is going to be a full blood moon!

Superstitious, I am not. Among my emergency medicine brothers and sisters, I am a rarity. During work, if I utter the words "all quiet," "silent," "simple, easy, slow," or any word or phrase that resembles a nice, reasonable working atmosphere, most of my colleagues will get upset and sometimes even threaten violence toward me. I can't blame them for their illusions and superstitious behavior. The hospital emergency department, or as most laymen like to call it, the emergency room (ER), is a strange place. This environment in which I have lived and worked as a board-certified emergency medicine physician is an emotional ride. The ride can take its passengers from excitement to nightmare in seconds. When you think you are disembarked and safe, you can be thrown back on. Within seconds, you are rolling higher and launching faster than the previous run. We picked this field as much to help people as we did for the exhilarating ride. What silly words I speak won't determine what kind of craziness might come through those doors.

However, tonight had something that transcends ominous worry and superstition. The staff will be freaked out by the full blood moon outside. Hell, ER shifts during regular full moons get some hospital staff jittery like alcoholics going into withdrawal. The meaning behind blood moons is something I won't share with my staff, but I will share it with you. The superstitious believe a blood moon brings chaos and disruption. Some people go so far as to believe one should not eat, should not have sex, and is not allowed to sleep until it is over. I say it is all a bunch of hogwash. The issue that might bring a rough shift is the fact tonight happens to be prom night. It was a warm, late-spring evening in May, with bedlam in the air. The statistics support increased alcohol consumption, sex among inexperienced teenagers, and other risky behavior. To make matters worse, both local high schools were holding prom on the same night. The schedulers apparently didn't communicate, so potential problems may multiply. Instead of spreading the craziness over two weekends as they usually do, we were going to get hit with it all on this most likely crazy Saturday night shift.

As I neared the hospital, a sense of foreboding hit me. I pulled into the hospital parking lot and looked around to assess the number of parked cars. *No more cars than a normal evening.* Sometimes my optimism overrides my realism. I remember thinking, *Tonight will be another uneventful shift with maybe one or two interesting encounters, but nothing to write home about.* I was about to turn off the ignition when the next song on the radio came on. "Bad Romance," Lady Gaga's latest chart-topping tune, started to play—ironic on a prom night. Contemplating sitting in my car through the entire song, I enjoyed one verse and then stepped out of my truck. Some would say I was tempting fate by not listening to the entire song. As you already know, I don't buy into unfounded fear. When my feet hit the black top, I could almost smell craziness in the air. Was I deluding myself about tonight's shift? *Oh no!* With prom and the expected full blood moon, anybody could find a reason to be especially stupid tonight. My stomach did a flip-flop as I looked into the sky and saw the sun's intensity was dwindling. The full moon was starting to be more apparent. In a couple hours, the reddish-brown color would be added. Instead of a signal like the Batman beacon bringing the cape crusader out to clean up the chaos, the reddish-brown flare of a bloody moon would be like an alert, signaling the evening mayhem to begin. A worrisome thought was lingering in my head as I walked into the emergency room entrance. Tonight, anybody who had ever drank alcohol or had sex was probably getting drunk and having sex, and of course, the prom boys and girls who had never drank alcohol before and were virgins were now on the verge of getting drunk and losing their virginity. What would this night shift bring? You are about to find out!

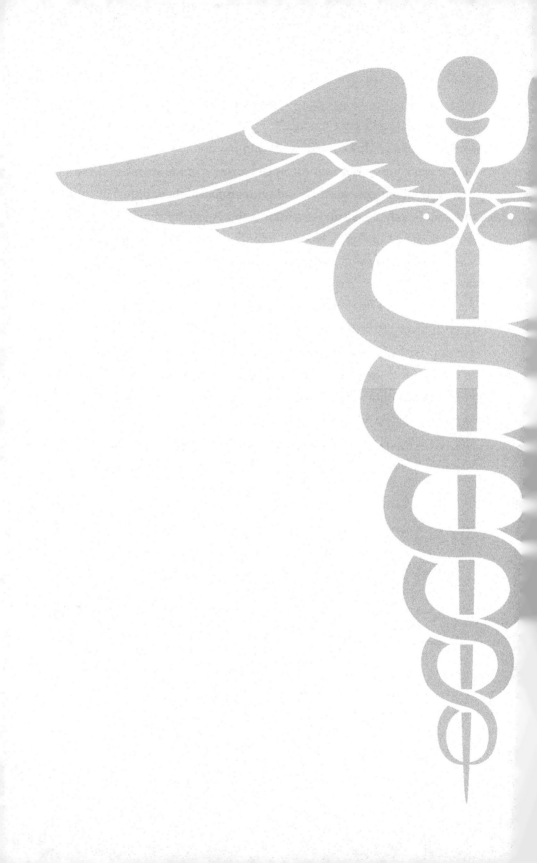

CHAPTER 1

Privates with Problems
5:54 p.m.

Walking into the emergency department, it only took a few seconds to assess the current climate. The ambient volume gives me a quick idea of how busy the department's current state might be. The combination of voices, monitors beeping, phones ringing, and people marching was currently at a normal level. I dropped off my lunch in the back-office fridge, hooked my stethoscope to the waist clip on my left hip, and greeted the morning doctor, who should be wrapping things up. My colleague, Dr. Jones, looked slightly tired, but not his usual ragged end-of-shift appearance. Like me, he doesn't wear a white lab coat but prefers our hospital-issued scrubs. Our navy blue scrubs have our names stenciled above the left breast pocket. We have two large pockets on our scrub pants. I keep utility scissors in my left pocket along with a few packaged tongue depressors.

Unlike Dr. Jones, I no longer wear a pager. My flip phone is left in my truck. I have yet to purchase what I've heard people call "smart phones." I was hesitant to embrace a phone that never leaves your side. During residency, I basically wore a pager 24/7. The pager ate with me, slept with me, went to the bathroom with me, and was two feet away when I showered. As a resident, I always had to be available as I spent time working in the operating room and intensive care unit in addition to my main location, the ED. However, as soon as the emergency medicine physician's residency ends, being on call is over. It's a sweet gig, being a doctor without having to take calls. Well, not having to take calls comes with a catch. The emergency departments are open 24/7. I exchange the no-call benefit for many night shifts, half my weekends, and sometimes over half my holidays. That is the price we pay for no calls. When I completed residency, that pager was the first thing I threw away. I hated being tied to that beeping contraption.

After twelve hours, I hoped to look as good as Dr. Jones after my coming shift. I was not thinking of his salt-and-pepper facial stubble that matches the hair on his head. It was his expression of contentment at finishing a solid day's work that I was focused on. Jones has twenty-plus years on me. He may not be able to move patients as quickly as I can, but he is not afraid to get bloody and work long hours. We both work more hours than the average emergency physician. I'm paying off school loans and still feel fresh, as I am only a few years out of residency. Unlike me, medicine is Dr. Jones' life, and most likely he will continue to work until he dies on a shift. Also, he figures if he works all the time, he won't make the mistake of marrying a fourth time and adding to his ever-mounting alimony bills he complains about on a daily basis.

"Hey, always nice to see you. It means I don't have to pick up any more charts," Jones greets me.

I respond by asking, "Anything you need to hand off? Let's see how quick we can get you out of here." Back then, we used to work single coverage. That means only one doctor is covering the entire ER. I wanted and loved independence. After finishing residency, where you work in an ED that has multiple doctors every single shift, I desired autonomy. I wanted complete ownership over the ED. The obligation for every single patient who walks, crawls, is carried in, or wheeled in is mine. The only problem was the number of patients coming into our ED was increasing each year. We had discussed switching from our then twelve-hour shifts to eight-hour ones. All of us thought we could handle the increasing volume and long hours. The department saw an average of sixty patients in twenty-four hours. That comes out to 2.5 patients an hour. Our volume for single coverage was nearing a tipping point, reason being that on busy days, like holiday weekends, we would see over ninety patients a day. At that volume of patients, we were exceeding what was considered a safe number of patients for one physician. We debated adding a mid-level practitioner, like a physician assistant (PA) or nurse practitioner (NP), specifically for the holiday weekends. This was nearly fifteen years before "quiet quitting" and the "great resignation." Even back then, it was impossible to get people to work holiday shifts that would be much more difficult than regular days, regardless of salary. However, masochist doctors will. In our group, I was the youngest and newest one of those. I would be damned if I would throw in the towel before my older partners. After all, more hours and busier shifts meant more money. I was fresh, fit, and could fly in the ER. Burn out was a long way off. *Wow, was I naive!*

"Hey, just a quick couple of discharges, and I should be out of here in five to ten minutes. I won't need to dump anything on you. I have a feeling my shift was the calm before the storm," Jones laughed as he hurried to his desk to finish up some charting. *Great!* I was glad about not getting any handoff patients. Hearing his opinion on the impending storm possibility—that part did not make me happy.

Let me explain what can occur at a shift change. When the ED is empty, the current doctor heads out when the other doc arrives. When the ED is not empty, some patients might be in the middle of their work up. For example, a patient presents with abdominal pain. After doing a history and physical, you realize they need more than a pain pill and an off-work note. The doctor orders IV (intravenous) fluids, blood tests, and an abdominal CT (computed tomography) scan. Let's say the CT scan has been ordered but not completed. Depending on the day, it could take another twenty minutes or possibly hours to get completed. Then, you still need to wait for the radiologist's read of the scan. If there is a surgical finding like appendicitis or a bowel abscess, now you throw in a phone call to the surgeon, additional medication orders, calls to inform the operating crew, etc., and soon the doctor finishing a twelve-hour shift finishes a fourteen-hour shift in no time. To limit working past shift change, we hand off the remaining patients to the new ER physician who recently arrived. Of course, the complicated patients bring even more confusion with handing off care. The disposition of patients is the key to being an efficient emergency medicine physician. When we encounter a patient, the choices are simple: admit, discharge, or transfer (there is always the option of sending them to the morgue, but today I'm pretty sure everybody makes it). Making the correct decision 100% of the time is the difficult part. When a medical provider encounters a patient part way through their care, often an accurate impression can be difficult to obtain. What did the patient look like when the initial doctor saw them? The patient looks comfortable now. Did the pain medication given an hour ago mask a serious issue? A normal lab reading may give the new doctor caring for a sick patient a false reassurance of a hidden life-threatening problem. Thankfully, Dr. Jones was finishing every patient he had already seen. Tonight, starting this shift, I was blessed to not have to deal with those issues. *How bad could tonight really be?*

I sat down at my desk to access the computer. A visual display of the emergency department layout had recently been installed. Our emergency department had twelve main beds and two observational beds in the back of the department. Our two large trauma rooms were partitioned by a wall, but in each room, only curtains separated the two individual beds, giving us four large main treatment rooms for our most critical folk. The nurses' and doctors' station was centered, with the four trauma beds on one side (rooms 1–4), the three monitored beds behind (rooms 5–7), and the remaining five beds on the opposite side from the trauma rooms (beds 8–12, plus 2 observational beds). Those five unmonitored rooms were mostly procedure rooms or rooms for low-acuity patients with urgent care complaints (casting, lacerations, and gynecological exams). Low acuity refers to less life-threatening complaints, and the patient is unlikely to be admitted in the hospital. Monitored rooms are used for higher-acuity cases. They have the ability to run continuous blood pressure, pulse oximetry, and heart rate and rhythm readings. In addition, they have space for multiple staff and added equipment to address any unstable patient needs.

The computer display gave a nice visual, but we were in its infancy and had yet to transfer to a completely digital department. We had recently begun getting lab results on the screen in addition to continuing our old paper lab printouts. Radiology would call every CT scan result during the day, and plain X-ray film results were scribbled on a piece of paper that was slipped into the X-ray film jacket. The ER doctors could trust the radiologist or inspect the X-rays themselves. Regular X-rays were still made on X-ray film and delivered to the doctor's desk in a large folder by the technician, or tech. This was vital because after 6:00 p.m., at the start of this shift, the ED doctors read all their own plain films. The radiologists would be in their cars by 6:00 p.m. and would overread all X-rays that had been taken after 6:00 p.m. the following morning. This gave the night doctor an extra responsibility. The CT results after 6:00 p.m. were delayed a bit. CT scans were sent to Australia, and a wide-awake radiologist across the ocean interpreted images and called us with a report on the phone. The computer X-ray reading stations had been installed, but we only used them

5

sparingly. None of us doctors wanted to rely exclusively on them yet. There is something about holding a film in the air, then bringing it to a patient's room and showing them the findings. The secretary would still type our lab and X-ray orders into their computer. The nurses' orders were still written on blue order sheets clipped to individual patient charts. The charts were numbered according to room numbers. To inform the nurses of new orders, we either used our voice or a color tag system. We would clip different colored tags to the chart clipboard: a red tag for medication orders, a blue tag for lab draws, and a black tag for a radiographic study. The age of the electronic medical record had yet to disrupt my future fully. Thus, I could still do my job without having to be glued to a computer screen. *Boy, how I miss those good old days.*

"Hey, Doc, here's your first patient of the night," the charge nurse giggled as she handed me a clipboard. My charge nurse for this shift was Sally. She was a few years my senior and very focused on doing a good job. Sally rarely giggled and never joked. She dressed nicely and was, I hate to say it, almost too professional. I always thought if she smiled more often and wasn't so serious, she would be more fun to work with. I reached for the chart as a loud, blood-curdling scream sounded through the entire department. As soon as the scream finished, the entire ED went silent. Only some faint beeping from a cardiac monitor could be heard. I couldn't tell if the scream came from a child or an adult or if they were a man or woman. All I could tell was it wasn't just physical pain that caused this scream; it also had a terror aspect, kind of like a person's worst nightmare had come to life. My nurse pointed at the chart in my hands, indicating the scream came from my first patient of the day. I looked down at the Room 9 clipboard; the chart read: CC: Junk caught in zipper, 18-year-old (y.o.) male

CC means chief complaint (the primary problem for which the person is seeking medical assistance). Ideally, it is the patient's stated problem verbatim; sometimes the triage nurse amends or makes an adjustment while typing, *for better or worse*).

Moving at breakneck speed, I place the clipboard on my desk. Usually I bring it into the exam rooms with me. I grab a bottle of lidocaine and a needle and syringe. In all honesty, I was at the patient's bedside in under thirty seconds. Many emergency medicine physicians gravitate toward this field because they are hyperactive. I am no exception, but I tend to be near or at the top on the hyperactive speed freak spectrum. Imagine a taller, less attractive Tom Cruise as your ER doctor—you get me? *I like to think so.* Mr. Cruise has some personality quirks that I share that are advantageous as an emergency medical physician. Yes, with the same intensity, and like the characters he portrays, I get the job done. Ok, like the legendary actor, I was probably too intense in my first decade or two as an emergency provider. However, I never received complaints in the "not timely" category. I am in the business of providing aid. The more painful the problem, the quicker aid was administered.

I enter Room 9. Sitting on the hospital bed is a shaking young white male wearing an all-red leather tuxedo with many gold necklaces around his neck. When I say white, I'm not only referring to his Caucasian race but also the extent of his complexion. He was ghost white, pale as fresh snow. This is a color that you obtain from fright, not blood loss (unless you are already dead). The red leather tuxedo and multiple gold necklaces would have been comical if he weren't gripping a blood-stained sheet that was covering his waist. The red leather was slightly darker than the bright red that was covering a small area of the white sheet. "I'm Dr. Adams. I'm going to take a look and at the same time numb things up, so in thirty seconds your pain will be gone." *Physical pain I can remedy near instanta-neously, but the psychological pain may take some time.* I lift up the sheet to access the true damage. Sensing his eyes are following me down toward his crotch, I stop inches before the big reveal. "Stop!" I firmly state. "I don't want you looking at it until I have it numbed up and you are feeling some relief. It hurts worse watching me inject the numbing medicine. Plus, do not move! You got it?" I finish by glaring straight into his eyes. This is one of those situations when the doctor needs to exert full control. Firstly, I don't want him flopping in bed, so I have to inject a moving target. Secondly, I remember his scream when I was thirty yards away, and now my ears are two feet from his mouth. My eardrums would not survive. He nods and reluctantly turns his head to face the wall. I lift the sheet to expose the entire scene. Some bloody, macerated tissue is interspersed in between a gold zipper that is either half drawn up or half drawn down, depending on your viewpoint. I'm not sure at this point if I'm looking at foreskin, glans, or shaft tissue. There is no active bleeding; only mild dried blood is par-tially obscuring the scene. Do you remember Ben Stiller's character from the movie *There's Something About Mary*? Most penises that are snagged in a zipper don't bleed much. The nurse hands me some iodine, and I pour it around the exposed skin. Back then, we put iodine on all wounds before we knew better. Prepping surrounding, non-injured tissue is the appropriate place for iodine cleansing. Iodine should not be placed on anything other than minor wounds and abrasions. Of course, my parents would douse my wounds with hydrogen peroxide, and many people still mistakenly con-tinue that practice. Hydrogen peroxide should not touch damaged tissue, period. Iodine is less toxic and a safer antiseptic. In reality, soap and water are really all that is necessary to treat almost every wound. My patient doesn't even move when the usually cold iodine liquid touches him. Most likely, the macerated tissue is no longer viable, and I will need to make sure my needle injects below the zipper area. I make the first injection on the top tissue above the zipper. Some anesthetic effect may travel below the zipper, and I also want to see if he jumps because of fear alone. "Oh! Doc, I felt something?" he questions. His eyes slowly turn from the wall toward the area I'm injecting. "Eyes on the wall, young man! The future of your family is in my hands," I order, while adding a little levity. Red tuxedo boy starts to sob quietly as Sally shakes her head. My attempt to bring a little humor falls flat. My other nurses would have found it funny. Sally's ultra-professionalism rears its no-fun head again. The second injection just below the zipper elicits a squeal of discomfort, but the red tuxedo boy bravely holds still. In all my years of injecting anesthetic agents, the most important thing for patients is not to move. Of course, not screaming is a close second. "Is it feeling numb?" I ask. "Doc, it doesn't hurt anymore," he answers.

Now that he is pain-free, I can attempt to remove the tissue from the zipper and ask him how this occurred. During my years, I have come to realize I practice differently than a few of my fellow doctors. I have over-heard some of my colleagues asking patients how they ended up hurting themselves before addressing the patient's pain. The obvious presentations don't need explanations. It blows my mind that some doctors delay pain relieving until they get all their questions answered. Early in my career, I adopted the approach of treating patients like I would want to be treated. In addition, I have found that after pain relief, patients give much more accurate explanations when pain is controlled or eliminated, especially when the exact narcotic dosage administered stops short of the uncon-scious line. As patients cross the border into la-la land, they become more forthright, almost as if they want to get everything off their chests and spill their guts. In addition to getting a better history, a more accurate physical exam is obtained. Of course, the patient needs much less narcotic dosage to obtain an accurate physical exam than the truth serum levels described above. A great example of this is when a patient has appendicitis. Many years ago, surgeons would advise emergency physicians not to administer pain medication to probable appendicitis patients until they had seen and pushed on those patients' abdomens. This was a sore point with many doctors working in the emergency setting and not wanting to wait for the surgeon before giving their patients some pain relief. Eventually, formal studies were done that proved better physical exams were obtained by both the ER doctor and surgeon after pain medicine had been given. Waiting to give pain medicine not only left your patient suffering longer, but it also decreased the accuracy of your physical exam. Of course, our current CT imaging is so accurate that these days we rely less and less on quality physical exams, but you didn't hear that from me. Well, maybe you did, because it's true.

Looking down after delivering the injection, I take in the area surrounding my patient's penile region. I noticed something pretty obvious that would have saved him this painful and costly hospital visit. "So do you not believe in underwear?" I ask him.

"Oh, Doc, my girl told me she would go to prom with me, and if I didn't wear underwear, she wouldn't either," he replies. Well, he might be regretting that now, but it would be hard not to agree to those terms as a dumb eighteen-year-old going to prom.

"What caused you to snare your penis in the zipper?" I finally ask.

"Well, Doc, my girlfriend was showing me what she had planned for when we got to the prom, and then she asked if I wanted a little before we left the house. I was busy watching her as I hurriedly pulled down my zipper, forgetting I was going commando, not paying enough attention, and I snagged my dick." While we were conversing, I had been unsuccessful in moving the zipper in any way, shape, or form. *This damn thing will not budge.* The tissue is so ensnared that my only hope is to remove the entire zipper and unclasp the actual zipper mechanism.

"Sorry, my man, but I'm going to cut out your entire zipper. I'll do it in a way that someone can restitch it back into your pants," I explain. His zipper appears to be actual gold, not painted gold. *Wonder what this young man's parents do?*

"Whatever you have to do, Doc. I just want to go home with my dick intact," he pleads.

"Your jewelry and gold zipper are impressive. Is your dad a famous rapper or something?" I ask.

"No, Doc. I like to spend my money on bling," he answers.

After spending another ten minutes without being able to detach the zipper mechanism, I decide to throw in the towel. I need to call my specialist, the urologist. Like all physicians, and specifically my fellow Emergency Medicine colleagues, we doctors have egos. We believe we can fix and solve most things that come through the door. We hate calling the specialists for little things that we should be able to handle. I have a gut feeling that this young man's penis is not the easy fix I initially thought it would be. "I'm going to call the urologist to see if he can get you unstuck," I say to my red tuxedo kid.

"Doc, what is a urologist?" he asks. His face is starting to show fear and panic again. His pale white cheeks have turned a healthier pinkish hue and are once again fading.

He had never heard of a urologist? To check his knowledge level, I ask him, "Have you heard of a gynecologist before?" I look at him.

"Of course. That's a pussy doctor, Doc!" he responds, slight concern still showing on his face. Inside, I laugh. Of course, teenage boys all know who a gynecologist is and will never see one, but they don't know what or who a urologist is. The irony is every man who lives a long life will eventually need to see the urologist.

"Well, simply put, the urologist is a dick doctor. We have a dick problem, so I'm calling in the specialist. I'll find out who is on tonight and see if they can come down and free your penis," I say as I walk out of his room. I ask my ED clerk, the person who covers the phones in the department, who my urologist is tonight. Tonight's clerk is Cindy, who is basically the secretary for all the ED employees. Like most of our ED clerks, Cindy is solid and knows her stuff. She is very professional, like Nurse Sally, but unlike Sally, she enjoys my attempts at humor.

"Doc, Dr. Richard Wang is tonight's on-call urologist," Cindy states. *So, Dick Wang is my dick doctor.* Pretty sure he has heard a few jokes about his name. You are probably wondering why I would risk the privacy of one of my fellow physicians by giving you his full name. Don't worry. This is the only physician in my recounting whose first and last name I will reveal. Why would I be so callous as to not protect a colleague's anonymity? Wang is the most common surname on the planet, and I have met three Dr. Richard Wangs. The two who went by Dick Wang were both urologists, and the one who went by Rich Wang was the neurosurgeon.

"Dr. Wang on line 2!" Cindy yells out.

"Hi Dick, this is Adams in the ED. I have a young man who got his penis stuck in his zipper. I wasn't able to detach the zipper, and it won't budge. I'm thinking the foreskin may need to go, and I figured I needed your expertise. He is in Room 9, all numbed up." I finish giving the pertinent details and wait for his response.

"Oh, I see. I get zipper detached. No problem. Be right down." The phone clicks out. *Great, I'll look inept at not getting the zipper to unclasp, but on the positive side, the kid might still make it to prom and not need a circumcision.*

I hear another chart fall into the to-be-seen rack. Turning my head, I see a mischievous smile on Nurse Betty's face. Pretty sure she is the one who placed said chart in the rack. I walk over to grab the new chart. Nurse Betty is waiting for me to catch her eyes. Betty is one of the few nurses who has seen a lot more than I have. Betty is old-school. She is professional, but unlike Sally, she enjoys all attempts at humor, preferring the off-colored jokes. She often sports classy makeup and wears more of the traditional scrubs. She is also a hard worker, so I have no problem when she has some fun at my expense. *She is being unusually tight-lipped, with no quick comment about my next patient.* Betty is usually very chatty and is great at giving me verbal updates throughout most shifts. Most of those verbal updates are quips about my inadequacies. Her silent treatment has me both curious and a bit worried. My guess is that she wants to see my reaction when I read this patient's chief complaint. Most likely, this means my second patient of the shift will be even more fun than patient number one. Giving Betty a quick smirk back, I grab the chart and look down at Clipboard Room 8: CC: F.B. in vagina 18 y.o. female

"Damn," I say. Betty starts giggling. FB is an abbreviation for foreign body. Unfortunately, two days ago I had back-to-back patients with the same complaint, and of course Betty was my nurse in both situations. This is a perfect example of why it is very important in emergency medicine to have a short memory. Why, you ask? If before each shift I recalled every blood curdling scream, every sobbing in despair patient, and some of the worst odors known to this world, who in their right mind would show up to work the next day? My two cases earlier in the week have left me a bit scarred. Especially when I see the exact same CC on this chart. One of those cases was a sad case of an alcoholic nearing menopause who left her tampon in for over a month. She presented feeling pelvic pain and having bad vaginal discharge. My nose has still not forgiven me for the stench that arose when I pulled that tampon out. The tampon both resembled and smelled like a dead mouse. Armed with only a surgical mask, I nearly lost my lunch to that seething vapor when that tampon cork was removed. (One benefit of the Covid pandemic is that N-95 masks are more readily available throughout the ED. The N-95 blocks a lot more odors than regular surgical masks.) My other patient was a young girl who was freaking out that she was going to die from toxic shock. She was convinced that the tampon she forgot to pull out before inserting a new one was going to kill her. I was able to retrieve the forgotten tampon and reassure her that toxic shock is rare, and in her case she didn't even have any signs of local infection. To lessen her fears, I casually shared the case I had seen earlier that same day. I described the poor woman's situation. It led to bad vaginitis, but it took over four weeks to develop. Even with all that, she was not in shock, and also went home doing fine.

As my mind was reliving the two similar encounters of the same chief complaint, Nurse Betty took some pity on me. "The foreign body is not a tampon," Betty smirked. "I wanted to see you squirm a little after what we went through earlier this week. It is a condom that fell off and the poor girl can't find it," Betty finished the explanation. I was more relieved that I wasn't dealing with another lost tampon than I was upset with Betty. She has a way of pushing people's buttons, yet not so much that they ever get that upset with her. In fact, most the ED staff would admit she lightens the atmosphere in the ED when it's needed most. Health care providers who have that skill are worth their weight in gold. I won't tell her that because it would go to her head. Betty doesn't need a larger ego.

"You could have saved me from dredging up those odiferous memories and typed, 'chief complaint: condom in vagina,' instead of 'foreign body,'" I plead.

"Where's the fun in that? Let's go fishing." Betty smiles as she leads the way to the patient's room.

"Hello," I call out as I knock on the door and turn the knob.

A faint voice responds, "Come in." Quickly, I scan the room. A young, red-cheeked brunette is on the exam table with a sheet covering her lower half, with a pink strapless prom dress pushed up near her lower abdomen. Sitting two feet away, trying and failing to melt into the wall, is an equally young boy wearing a bright blue tuxedo.

"Hi, I am Dr. Adams, and you already know Nurse Betty here. Let's see how quickly we can get your problem solved so you two can enjoy the rest of prom night." The young lady stares daggers at the blue tuxedo boy. If looks could kill, he'd be far too dead for me to resuscitate. Obviously, neither of these two has any intentions of enjoying the rest of prom night. Based on my prior experience not only as a doctor, but I reluctantly admit, as a horny young man, I sincerely doubt this sniveling blue tuxedo boy was ever wearing a condom. Staring straight at the blue tuxedo boy, I reached down for my most intimidating scary voice. I try to recall the wizard, Gandalf, from the Lord of the Rings, when he grew in size and stature trying to talk sense into Bilbo. "I have to ask that everybody be honest. Are you 100 percent sure you had a condom on when having sex?" I continue to glare at the blue tuxedo boy.

He starts to shake slightly and slowly his mouth opens. Before he utters a single syllable, the young girl screams out, "Of course he was wearing a condom! I put it on him myself. No way am I getting pregnant the first time I ever have sex." Her venom eyes shift quickly from blue tuxedo boy to me and back to tuxedo boy. *Damn this boy picked a firecracker and she is far from finished exploding.*

"Sorry. I don't want to put you through an unneeded procedure," I respond. Nurse Betty starts to position the young lady in the stirrups and hands me a disposable plastic speculum with battery attachment. Truthfully, I don't want to do a pelvic exam on a pissed-off teen who ended up in the emergency department hours after losing her virginity. To point out a personal feeling, vaginal exams are one of the worst parts of my job. Ok, it isn't at the top of the list. That would be telling family members a loved one has died or soon will. But it's right up there. The majority of women don't want a stranger up in their business, so to speak. Then, you specifically take a moment in time when they are either in pain or experiencing a stressful health crisis and some strange dude is poking his hands and cold plastic (not that long ago it was cold metal) into their anatomically most sensitive area of their entire body. To make it even worse, a high percentage of my pelvic exams come from a particular subset of the population—young women who have never had a pelvic exam before. They have either not yet become sexually active or have just recently started having sex before a pelvic problem forced them to the ED. I have to do their first ever vaginal/pelvic exam. *Boy oh boy, sign me up for that. Sounds like fun. If you are a rapist.* During a busy emergency department, I try to be quick and efficient with all my interactions and examinations, especially the exams that are, shall I say, more uncomfortable than the others. As I have said before, I am very quick. I am capable of doing a rectal exam in seconds, but rushing the placing of a vaginal speculum and performing an up-tempo pelvic exam is not advisable. Thus, it is not something that is done in a flash.

I switch on the battery pack that is attached at the base of the speculum and now I have a light. Quickly, I scan her labia, hoping unrealistically the condom got hidden in pubic hair. Surprisingly, she is clean shaven—no hair, or even any stubble. Of course, there was no condom in sight. *I couldn't be so lucky.* I grab a small portion of lube for the speculum, knowing that too much lube will interfere with my finger sensation if the speculum exam is unsuccessful. Conversely, I know she will need enough lube for the speculum not to hurt or possibly tear her. The speculum now in and fully expanded, I scan intensely, hoping to see any piece of the condom. I am looking for any shiny, dull, or mismatched discolored area. No luck.

After what seems like a while for me and an eternity for her, I give up the visual inspection. I gently retract the speculum and remove it. The girl lets out a sigh and then resumes her glaring toward the blue tuxedo boy. Betty assists by adding her pair of eyes, burrowing hatred toward the tuxedo boy. If he were a dog, his tail would be tucked up tight between his legs right now. *I almost feel bad for him if he turns out to be innocent.* "Well, I was hoping we could see it, but usually we have to find it by feel," I regretfully inform. The term "we" really refers to me, but I am trying to make a conscious effort to make this sound more like a team approach. I slowly insert two fingers and begin to palpate around her entire pelvic area. I cover the entire right side then left side, making sure I don't miss any spots, while trying to be both quick and thorough at the same time. I feel nothing unusual and start wondering if the blue tuxedo boy pulled a fast one. There is another blaring fact adding to my opinion that he might have pulled the condom off before engaging in said activity. This particular exam room is very chilly and both the young prom woman and I have yet to break a sweat. She and I are the ones exerting. Blue tuxedo boy is not only sweating, water is dripping off of him. He is perspiring so profusely the sprinkling sweat is forming small pools on the floor. I gently remove my fingers and concede. I hate giving up, especially when it comes to removing foreign bodies from patients. I usually pride myself by having great success at finding and removing objects that are both easily seen or seriously hidden inside my patient's bodies. *Damn it, this might not be my failure, as the blue tuxedo boy could still be the culprit. I'll try a different approach and see if the blue tuxedo boy comes clean.* "I'm going to call the gynecology doctor on call and have him see if he can find what I am not able to," I state. Looking down on the sweaty, shifty-eyed blue tuxedo boy, I give him one last fierce glare. I'm doing my best impression of his pissed off one day lover. He doesn't move, but avoids my eyes and looks to the exam bed as his prom date removes her feet from the stirrups. Betty slowly lets go of the young woman's hand so she can cover herself up. The poor girl extends the white sheet to cover her entire waist and lower extremities, trying to regain some modesty and any remnant of control. I feel bad for her, but also for my failure. *I did not solve her problem. I take a second to forgo my ego and put my patient's feelings first. Damn, the perturbed girl might not even be half way through her ED prom disaster.* The gynecologist might do an exam and possibly an ultrasound (US) study. At this point, I'm going to let the specialist decide the next course of action.

I step out and ask Cindy to call the gynecologist on call. She says she'll do it and informs me Dr. Wang has been in Room 9 for a long while now. *Great, maybe he was successful in taking care of the zipper boy's penis problem. Dammit, I'm 0 for 2 to start my shift.* I walk over to Exam Room 9 and right before I knock on the door, it opens. An exasperated Dr. Wang emerges. "I unable to get penis unstuck. Damn zipper can't disconnect. I take red leather bling boy to OR. He getting snip snip, circumcision," Dr. Wang laughs while he skips out of the emergency department. I hear him humming to himself as his feet glide to and fro in a rhythmic pattern across the outdated tile floor that should have been replaced a decade ago.

"Doctor, you're needed in Room 5. Now! I punched in early when I saw him come through the waiting room," Nurse Melody yells. Melody's shift must start at 7PM. She is one of my rookie nurses who is surprisingly quick. Surprising, not because she is new and inexperienced, but because she is eight months pregnant and plans to work until she goes into labor. *I pray I'm not working that shift.* I'm not a big fan of delivering babies. I am quickly pulled away from the humorous image of the urologist who truly loves his job. I bolt to Room 5 and see a pale young man covered in blood from the waist down. A nurse is hooking him up to the monitor and Sally is starting an IV. He can't be much older than 20, but unlike my earlier penile bleeder, this guy's paleness is from massive blood loss. "Where is the source of the bleeding? Is this a gunshot wound? I didn't know we had a Rig out!" I blurt as I'm grabbing a gown and gloves.

"It's my butthole that's bleeding," the patient responds much more calmly than I.

Melody looks over to the corner of the room and asks, "Who shot you in the butthole?" I finish grabbing some gauze and follow the direction of Melody's gaze to a petite young girl standing in the corner of the room. I had not even noticed her and I am usually pretty perceptive of my surroundings. She looks barely sixteen years old, and probably weighs around eighty-five pounds. She is wearing a small, revealing pink tank top that shows much more cleavage than any girl her frame should possess. She has tiny tight shorts and nothing else. The most alarming feature of this tiny woman, if she is indeed old enough to be called a woman, is that the lower half of her body is completely coated in blood. Her shorts have some blood stains, but from her upper thighs to her toes her natural skin color is completely obscured by a thin layer of dark dried blood. I turn to Nurse Betty. "Call the blood bank and tell them to emergency release four units of packed red blood cells now. Get a second IV and start 2 liters of normal saline wide open. What is his pressure?" I finish. I look up to monitor and see 60 systolic before anybody can answer me. *Bloody shit! This is serious. I need to act quickly!* "What happened Mr…" I realize I have no idea what his name is, and right now it doesn't matter.

"Um, my girlfriend was pegging me with a strap on a little too rough," my pale patient mutters as he tried to stay conscious. *He is bleeding out from probably an underage girl giving him anal sex.*

"Let's roll him on his belly," I inform the nurses. "Clench your anus until I tell you to relax," I order the patient.

My patient starts muttering, "It's not her fault. I told her to do me as hard as she could. Oh, I feel dizzy. So, she unstrapped and held it in her hand, going as har…."

"Whoa! I got the picture. How long ago was this?" I cut him off and ask.

"I remember feeling the tearing before blood erupted. Blood kept coming, so I sat on the toilet awhile. Maybe four hours ago. She kept telling me, 'We need to go to the ER,'" my patient finishes with a mild moan. *His embarrassment postponed him from seeking medical help. I won't tell him that in reality most of the staff won't even remember his name two hours from now, if they ever knew it to begin with.* I finish hooking up suction and point to a bunch of gauze boxes filled with 4 x 4s. Melody hands me the box. I opened the small box of gauze pads.

"I need at least three more of these boxes," I say to no one in partic-ular. *I take in his story along with combining the images of his female sexual accomplice and the image of his lower torso. I can't help but picture a volcano erupting. The initial event often is a huge explosion of force upwards followed soon by flowing lava in various amounts that originate from the starting source. It is a natural occurrence with violent, often deadly consequences. It is kind of like rough sex gone horrible.*

My patient, now laying naked on his belly, is clenching so tight he is shaking from the effort. *He will soon fatigue and won't be of any help.* "Don't unclench, but relax a little. I want you to clench your anus at an effort that you could hold for 30 minutes if you had to," I instruct. He stops shaking, but some bright blood starts dribbling from his gluteal fold. I instruct Melody that I will need her to slowly spread the patient's butt cheeks. I grab the suction in one hand and some gauze in the other, and tell my patient to slowly unclench. At the same time, I instruct Melody to open his cheeks wide. His entire butt and posterior surface is caked in blood. I place suction near his anus. I need to see if this opening is close enough that I can suture here in the emergency department, or if he has to go to the operating room. I get visualization for a split second before blood covers the area too fast for suction to keep clear. There is no tear at the anal entrance and nothing slightly shallow. "Shit! it's deep," I accidentally say out loud. Blood continues to ooze steadily, but after turning suction to maximum I have just enough to keep pace so that I have good visibility on the surface. It isn't gushing, but continues with a steady trickle. I motion Melody to move her hands further towards his anal opening and spread more forcefully. "Somebody turn on the overhead light and position it right above my suction catheter," I instruct. Hovering nearby is a fully gowned up Sally, who is always present for whatever is needed. Loudly projecting my voice at the patient, I order, "Clench tight again, I'm going to suction a little ways in to see if I can locate the tear and see how big it is." I continue to suction the area pretty clean and am pleasantly surprised how wide his anal opening actually has become, as to allow pretty good lower area visualization. "Slowly unclench," I tell him as I have the suction catheter many inches down into his rectal vault. Oozing returns steadily, but not before I am able to visualize a large portion of the tear. I pack in as many gauze 4x4s as I can and then tell him to clench again for the long term. "I want the strongest effort you can maintain for another 30 minutes. The tear is at least one inch long (*probably much longer*) and will need to be fixed in the operating room. Betty, tell Cindy to get me the surgeon on the line, and start transfusing as soon as the blood arrives," I comment.

"Hey Doc, blood bank has arrived and is carrying the blood right behind you and so is the surgeon. I called him as soon as I saw how much blood was on the patient and his girlfriend," Betty responds in a matter-of-fact manner. Nurses who not only know their stuff, but take initiative are worth their weight in gold. I'm pretty sure I made a similar comment like that before. Well, the bottom line is, all great nurses are worth their weight in gold.

I make eye contact with my surgeon. I quickly tell him of the anal findings I recently discovered. My surgeon leans over the patient and whispers into his ear. I try to catch a few of the words when Cindy peeks her head into Exam Room 5 and says, "Dr. A, Big John on Line 2 returning your call regarding the girl in Treatment Room 8." Cindy had left her desk and poked her head into the chaos to inform me. Understandably, she has an opportunity to be helpful and maybe witness some of the action involving one of the more exciting patient encounters. Answering phones and directing calls is a thankless but crucial job. It also can appear rather dull, but certainly not when you compare it to other secretarial jobs on the planet, especially when you see doctors and nurses wearing gowns soaked in blood and running around like circus performers within ten feet from where you sit every day. Cindy has a vital job, but probably the only job in the department that has no direct patient contact. I can't blame her if she wants to witness the end result of a tiny woman nearly killing a man by strap on.

Speaking of damage to a person's private region, I go to speak to my on-call gynecologist. *Of all the luck, my poor deflowered prom girl gets Big John, the nicest doctor known to humankind.* Unfortunately, he is also the largest doctor I have ever met, hence the nickname Big John. Imagine if you will if NBA legend Shaquille O'Neal was a white gynecologist. You would be picturing Big John. Yes, probably like Shaq, he can pick up a basketball with only his index finger and thumb. *Not the size of hands you want in your daughter's vagina, or wife's for that matter.* I pick up Line 2. "Hey John, it's Adams in the ED. Have a kinda sad case of a possible condom in a young girl's vagina. She decided to lose her virginity before going to prom. She put the condom on the boy and they lost it. I was not able to find it. *I start picturing Big John doing a manual vaginal exam with hands the size of tennis rackets. The poor girl will never want to have sex again. I need to try and limit her damage.* You want me to order an ultrasound? No, you don't? Ok. You're going to check yourself? Oh, ok. See ya soon," I hung up. *Damn, I tried!* I'll tell Betty to offer her 1 mg (milligram) of Ativan before Big John arrives. *Slight sedation could help as I am fearful that the unlucky girl started the day with a virgin vagina, but may end the day with one that resembles a porn star.*

I walk back toward my rectal bleeding patient's room as the surgeon walks out to speak to me. The surgeon is laughing as he sits down at my desk. Before he picks up the phone, he turns to me. I was surprised to see him alone, as this month he has a surgical resident and medical student following him, along with his usual PA. So, I ask, "Hey, where is your entourage?"

He responds, "Oh, I gave them a night off as I'm treating them all to the hospital golf tourney Sunday. I want them rested, but I'll still have them rounding super early in the morning, so hopefully I can sleep in. They will be bummed to miss this case. Hah! I said bummed. I'm going to call the OR and we'll take him right up. Now that the blood is hung, his BP is holding. That young man will most likely have a colostomy bag for the summer. Adams, they told me that tiny girl in there is the one who tore his ass up. Man, she looks like jailbait to me. Gotta love prom night." My surgeon continues chuckling as he picks up the phone to dial the OR.

I look down at my watch. 18:52 hours. *Oh man, my night is not even one hour in. Three patients and three calls to specialists with two going to the operating room. Wow, if I keep up this pace for eleven more hours, I'll leave here looking as bad as my patients.* Before I can wallow in my misery, a large shadow descends over me. At six foot two inches, I rarely have to look up to people. Granted my patients are usually lying supine in hospital beds. Also, most nurses and doctors are shorter than me. Big John was the exception. In addition to his massive size was his contagious smile and ability to never get ruffled. His mannerisms leaned a bit toward the feminine side, which made him much more comforting as a gynecologist/obstetrician.

"Adams, what room is this young girl with the foreign body?" John politely asks.

"Room 8. I'll introduce you," I respond. Walking over to Room 8's door, I knock and reach for the handle. I momentarily hesitate about accompanying him, but I want to see if he has a better inspection technique than me. Truthfully, I didn't want to watch her go through an exam again, but if Big John found that condom while I was hiding at my desk, I'd feel like such a scrub. We walk in and the young girl's eyes bug out to the size of dinner plates as her lips start to quiver with fear. Blue tuxedo dude's entire body starts to tremble like he is going to be probed, not her. "This is our gyn doc on call…"

"Hi, you can call me Dr. John." Big John interrupts me with his words as his gentle reassuring smile spreads across his face. Nurse Betty once again helps the young lady get into position and holds her hand.

"Doc, she just refused the sublingual Ativan," Betty informs me.

Well, she had sex with a blue tuxedo dweeb boy, why start making good decisions now? I cringe during the exam, and feel as if everybody but Big John is holding their breath. In actuality, the patient was holding her breath throughout the entire exam. Good thing for her though, Big John finished quickly and efficiently. Dr. John steps back with an empty hand, "There is no condom in there young lady." John confirms my thoughts. In my medical experience, a broken condom can happen, but a lost condom is like the mythical unicorn. It might have existed, but in reality neither the yearning young woman nor the ER doctor will ever find one.

My ego is intact, but I feel terrible for what the poor girl has just gone through. Nurse Betty hands the girl some tissues to wipe tears from her eyes and few more down below. Dr. John turns to walk out. "Step outside with us," I state as I look blue tuxedo boy straight in the eyes. Begrudgingly he stands up and I let him walk out in front of me, a few steps behind Big John. I close the door behind me. I dwarf blue tuxedo boy similar to how Big John towers over me. I look up at Big John, then down to the quaking little man child. Big John cracks his knuckles and it sounds like a thunderstorm. "Tell the truth!" John and I say simultaneously.

Tuxedo boy starts to stammer, "Umm, I took it off right after she put it on, but after I had her turn around." John and I look at each other slightly confused.

"Go on," I order him.

"I told her the doggie style is easiest for the first time, so I could remove the condom without her knowing. I threw it in the far corner of the room as soon as she turned around. I threw it so far that she wouldn't see it after I was finished," he stopped.

Big John's face was getting red and he took one step toward the blue tuxedo boy. John's chest was now at the boy's head level. *I didn't want John to get in trouble for losing his cool on this shady kid. But I did want this condom magician to get some sort of beating.* "Get your ass back in that room and you tell her the entire truth, now!" I yell. He tries to walk past me toward the exit, but Big John grabs his collar, opens the door, and firmly places him back in the room.

"Tell her now!" John says so softly that it was way scarier than when I yelled. John closes the door behind him as he mumbles, "We'll be listening outside." As the door closed, I looked up to John and saw his face slowly resume a normal hue. We stand silent, nearly pressing our ears to the door. We hear him give a quick confession, then she erupts like Mount St. Helens.

"YOU WHAT? YOU FUCKIN PIECE OF SHIT! GET OUT! I NEVER WANT TO SEE YOUR STUPID ASS FACE EVER AGAIN!" That was when Big John reaches down and grips the doorknob tight. She continues yelling as I see John's grip get a little tighter. "I TOLD YOU TO LEAVE!"

Crashing sounds start coming from the room in addition to, "The doorknob won't turn, ouch stop throwing things, I'm trying to leave."

"Think he's had enough?" John asks me.

"No, but I don't want that little delinquent as a new patient either. You better let go before she gives him a real injury if she hasn't already," I snicker. John lets go of the doorknob and the door bolts open. Blue tuxedo boy looks at us and sprints down the hall much faster than I would have guessed he was capable of. Nurse Betty walks out of the room covering her ears and staring at Big John and me. We had forgotten she was still in there. "Sorry, Betty!" We both apologize. Betty smiles as she continues rubbing her ears, accessing if any permanent damage was done by all the yelling.

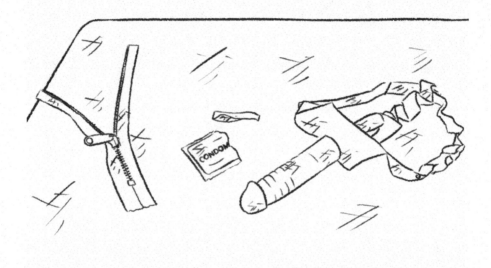

I felt bad for Betty, but what the poor young woman experienced was dreadful. Today's events will most likely leave a scar over all her sexual activity in the future. I have an idea that may help this young woman's future sexual experiences. Maybe we can influence her to make decisions that put her in the more dominant position. Giving control back to someone who's only sexual experience was tainted might be the best way I can help this young woman. "Betty, I have a favor to ask that may aid our young female patient. You saw the blood covered girl who caused Room 5's backdoor injury?" Betty nods. "She needs some cleaning and clothes and then someone to bring her to the operating waiting room. I was wondering if you wouldn't mind introducing her to our recently tricked young lady who Big John and I both examined. See if you can encourage strap-on girl to share the details relating to what might be a more empowering life's motto: IT IS BETTER TO GIVE THAN TO RECEIVE!"

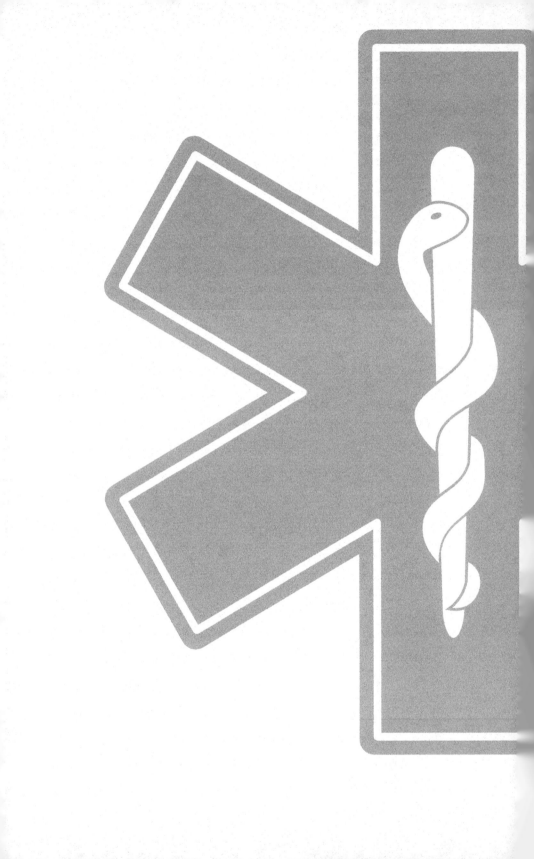

CHAPTER 2

Respect the Sex Organs
7:17 p.m.

"Doctor, an ambulance is pulling in with a seizure patient. We'll take him into Treatment Room 2. The medics sound rattled. We didn't respond to their first call and the patient didn't stop seizing until after they gave him a third benzo," Nurse Sally reports to me.

"Thanks. Turn up the EMS radio. The damn thing is either too quiet or way too loud, but we can't afford to miss calls. I'll meet them at the ambulance bay," I reply. Usually, seizure patients are very straight forward. Witnessing someone seize is alarming, but the majority of the time it is far from life threatening. Over one percent of adults have epilepsy. In addition, up to five percent of children will experience a febrile seizure and an equal percentage of alcoholics will have a withdrawal seizure sometime during their life. Paramedics, like most emergency medical workers, usually get a bit desensitized to seizing patients. *I wonder why they are rattled?*

I meet the two paramedics at our now open large entrance doors. The ambulance bay is a ramp covered entrance that opens up smack dab in the middle of our department right in front of the main desks. In seconds, we can wheel a gurney into one of our large trauma rooms. Both medics look frazzled. This is the final run of the day for Kim and Dan. The paramedics do 12 hour shifts like I do, as do most of the nurses. Their foreheads are dripping sweat. "Give me the low down!" I ask, looking down at the patient. I don't wait for a response as I do a quick sternal rub and see if I get any response to the inflicted painful stimuli. Nothing! He is a large adult male probably around thirty years old, roughly six foot and little over two hundred pounds.

"Well, Doc, he and his girlfriend just finished having sex when he grabbed his head and started seizing. He only stopped when we pulled up, after already giving IV Ativan, Valium, and Versed," Kim answered.

Damn! "No past seizure history? How long total before he stopped seizing? Girlfriend on the way?" I ask. I have an annoying habit of blurting out multiple questions before the first question is answered.

"No prior seizures Doc. Um she said he was shaking non-stop for possibly thirty minutes before we got there and another 20 minutes in route." *Witnesses over estimate seizure time unless they actually time it with a watch, but this patient's duration is extreme.* "She was right behind us driving as fast as Dan," answers Kim, referring to her partner, who usually drives like a bat out of hell. *They both understand that this is a rare life-threatening seizure patient. Now I know why they were rattled. This was not a simple recurrent or withdrawal seizure.* This patient was in severe status epilepticus. Status epilepticus is a seizure over five minutes or multiple seizures in a five minute period without returning to normal level of consciousness between episodes. This patient is critical and I have to find out the cause and stop the seizures from continuing.

The nurses are hooking him to the monitor as I start spouting off orders. "Tell respiratory to get down here with a vent and tell CT I want a head CT as soon as I am done intubating. Also, I want both Dilantin and Versed drips started, full labs, and drug screen. Sally throw in a quick foley," I order. The first thing to do with an unstable patient is to stabilize.

Looking at the monitor, I am pleasantly surprised to see a stable blood pressure and an understandably fast heart rate. In the ER, we keep it simple and focus on the ABCs—airway, breathing, and circulation. Having a good blood pressure and solid heart rate establishes the C, or circulation. I need to start at the beginning or A, the patient's airway. A seizing patient can aspirate or as in this particular case and his extended seizure duration, could stop breathing all together. I need to protect this patient's airway. Intubating a patient refers to placing a tube into the trachea to provide artificial ventilation. Once the tube is placed, we can use a bag that's connected to an oxygen source that a person has to manually squeeze or use a ventilator unit that works hands free once we set in certain parameters. The medications I ordered are anti-seizure drugs, as I need to make sure his seizure activity doesn't return. While all this is going on, my brain is working out possible causes or etiologies for his seizure. I need to know why he is seizing before I can provide a definitive treatment. The one glaring possibility that tops my differential diagnosis list is terrible. An acute brain bleed can present as a new onset seizure, especially severe status type. In fact, one of the most famous emergency medicine board questions described a young male patient with the sudden worst headache of life after masturbating. What is the likely diagnosis? The answer is a subarachnoid hemorrhage! The exertion act causes an unknown brain aneurysm to rupture. The brain bleeding then causes the seizure. My patient was having sex and grabbed his head before his seizure started. *Shit! People joke about kicking the bucket while having sex, but not at thirty years old.*

I am at the head of the bed and instruct my nurse to give some IV Succinylcholine, a neuromuscular blocker, the fancy name for a paralytic medicine. Waiting for him to become completely paralyzed, I am standing armed with an endotracheal (ET) tube and a laryngoscope. A laryngoscope is a metal device that allows visual inspection of the vocal cords to allow proper placement of the ET or breathing tube. In almost all emergency departments today, the old metal laryngoscopes are collecting dust as plastic fiber optic ones with high quality anti-fog cameras allowing a monitored perfect anatomical close-up picture have replaced the old standbys. I easily position the laryngoscope with my left hand, and with my right hand begin to slide the ET tube through the visualized vocal cords. Suddenly, my patient starts seizing again. Leaving the ET tube in place, I retract the laryngoscope seconds before his teeth clench, saving him a mouth full of chipped teeth. His entire body is convulsing and I am about to yell at my nurses for being too slow with the anti-seizure drugs. Lucky for me, I looked up and saw the hanging IV medications before opening my big mouth and trying to lay blame where it didn't belong. Both Dilantin and Versed drips are not only hung, but dripping into the patient's nice flowing IV line. *What the hell is going on?* Most seizures will stop after giving anti-seizure medication. The few exceptions will stop after adding a second medicine. This patient has had four medications that usually terminate seizures often by themselves. "Give him 10 mg of Vecuronium or 100 mg of Rocuronium, whichever one is in the intubation med tray," I order. Those are two longer acting paralyzing medications.

With the patient intubated, we now have a secure airway and provide the breathing for the patient. A and B of the airway and breathing checklist are completed. Now I can focus on how to abate the seizure activity. Also, I need to get him to CT and don't want an inaccurate study because of movement. As soon as the Rocuronium hits his vein, he stops shaking. Everybody in the room lets out a long breath. "Quickly, take a chest X-ray and let's get him into CT. Oh, set up a lumbar puncture (LP) tray at bedside for his return," I say to everybody, failing to suppress my anxiety. If a brain bleed is seen on CT, I won't need to do the lumbar puncture. However, if the CT is negative, the lumbar puncture will be needed for multiple reasons.

A small percentage of subarachnoid hemorrhages (SAH) can be missed on CT, but diagnosed with lumbar puncture. Also, infection or other neurologic disorders can be deduced from cerebrospinal fluid (CSF). The lumbar puncture, or layman's spinal tap, is not as scary or painful as people fear. It is a simple procedure of obtaining CSF from the low back. Patients often are placed on their side, a small lumbar area is numbed up, and a hollow needle is inserted to obtain CSF. I have mixed feelings about wanting the CT to give me the answer. If it gives me the answer, my job becomes easier but at the patient's expense. An aneurysmal brain bleed has poor prognosis. If negative, I may find a less ominous cause, but the investigation will be far from over. The CT scan goes smoothly and I call the radiologist to read the images as soon as possible. "Radiologist on line 1!" somebody yelled. I grab the phone, "Hey it's Adams, anything on the head CT?" The radiologist on the other end of the line gives me an all clear, completely negative scan report. *Great! But what is causing his seizures then?* My patient dodged a deadly bullet. Now I need to do my best Sherlock Holmes impersonation. Unlike the medical shows that frequently depict multiple diagnostic dilemma patients, they are not an everyday occurrence. During an entire shift, the ER doctor probably sees only one case that is actually rare or difficult to diagnose. We call the rare cases zebras. In comparison, most cases that present to the ER are horses. If you drove around the country avoiding zoos, how many zebras would you see? On that same drive how many horses would you see? You get the point.

My initial diagnosis is probably wrong, and that is a good thing. However, I now have to do the lumbar puncture and continue searching for answers. "Doctor, he is seizing again!" Betty yells.

"Shit! Repeat the Rocuronium! Also, give him two grams of IV Rocephin; *If this is infectious, I've already delayed treatment too long.* Let's

35

do the LP, then I need to talk to his girlfriend!" The Rocuronium does its job and the patient remains paralyzed, allowing me to perform the LP without any issues. A moving target is no fun, but also increases an inaccurate CSF sample, which could compromise the results. Luckily, the CSF was completely clear, ruling out bleeding and also decreasing the chance for infections like meningitis or encephalitis. The CSF is still sent to the lab looking at glucose, protein, cell count levels, and still accessing for any organisms. My top differential diagnosis is now pointing toward a drug induced etiology. Meningitis or encephalitis infection diagnoses are still a possibility. Usually, one tube of CSF is held in the lab in case the doctor decides to add further testing like viral cultures. Other possibilities I can't discount: undiagnosed epilepsy, repetitive sounds or flashes exposure, metabolic-like electrolyte deficiencies, or head injury that did not show up on CT. The issue that has me confused and stressed is that all the listed seizure causes usually stop seizing with much less IV treatment.

"Doc, this is his girlfriend, Becca," Betty states as she escorts a scared, young, red-haired beauty into the room. Becca is tightly clutching the cloth belt that is holding her satin red robe securely around her body.

"Becca have a seat. I'm Dr. Adams and I need to ask you some questions. It is really important that you answer everything honestly."

"Ok," she responds.

I begin, "Does your boyfriend take any drugs?" Becca shakes her head side to side. "I won't tell the police and I won't judge. I really need to know if he has taken anything." She shakes her head again, indicating no. "Becca, he didn't inject, snort, inhale, or swallow anything?" I was desperate to find any straw to grasp onto.

"No, nothing! He doesn't even like me smoking pot," Becca responds and begins crying.

"Ok, did he have any recent travel, cold symptoms, sick contacts, anything at all?" I ask.

"No, he was feeling fine until after our second time we had sex," Becca answers.

"Dr. Adams, CBC, comp all normal, understandably an elevated CK" Sally reports. *That rules out electrolyte or sugar issues being the culprit.* I continue grilling Becca for answers, "How many times did you have sex today?" I wasn't sure if the number of times he had sex would help me find out why he was seizing, but it was an obscure path that I was hoping would lead somewhere helpful.

"Well, we are trying to get pregnant and I am ovulating, so we planned to have sex all weekend long," Becca responds. I tell her to continue. "Well, after he finished the second time, he complained of a little headache and dizziness. He never gets headaches. So, I was a little worried. He took a little rest before we went at it a third time and I could tell he wasn't feeling right," Becca says, wiping her tears away and then reaching down toward her crotch area. I watched her rearrange the red robe that had bunched up near her pelvis. She started scratching between her legs.

"What do you mean he wasn't feeling right? Why are you scratching…?"

"Doctor we have a chest pain patient in 4, here is his EKG, they're putting in an IV now," Nurse Betty hands me the EKG and runs back towards Room 4. I look down and see the electrocardiogram (ECG or EKG) showing a ST Elevation Myocardial Infarction (STEMI). Myocardial Infarction (MI) is the medical terminology for heart attack. An EKG has a particular area that is called the ST segment. When this area is elevated, it often corresponds to a heart attack, coronary blockage, in the particular cardiac area represented by that ST segment. My new patient, who I had yet to see, was most likely having a heart attack.

"Excuse me Becca. Sally, let me know if his status changes and if the drug screen shows any abnormalities when it results."

I enter Room 4 and see a middle-aged man, slightly ashen color, sweaty black head of hair with silver streaks at the sides. The EKG electrodes placed on his exposed chest looked like small plastic animals in a black forest of deep chest hair. When I get closer I see the nurses had to shave his chest in order for the electrodes to gain connection. The chest hair was like a black fur blanket. My guess is that shaving down to the skin must have taken a while. I look at the monitor: Blood pressure (BP): 170/95 Heart Rate: 95 Pulse Ox: 99%. Rhythm is sinus and regular.

"Hi, I'm Dr. Adams, (I look down at the EKG for my patient's name, usually printed at top) Mr. Thompson. Describe to me what you are currently feeling in your chest," I instruct.

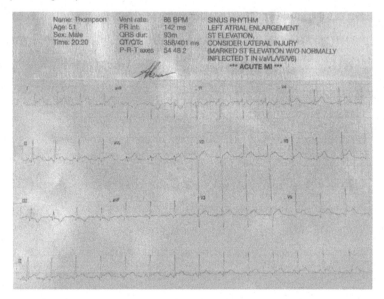

"Um, a slight pressure but not as bad as it was. It's just slightly annoying now, not terrible like earlier," Mr. Thompson explains.

"When did the pain start and what were you doing at the time?" I ask.

"Oh, probably about an hour ago and um we were, um…" He was having difficulty answering the rest of my question when I noticed a red-headed woman sitting nearby in a red silky robe. A wave of deja vu hit me. She was older than Becca, my seizure patient's girlfriend. But like Becca, she must have been in her birthday suit when the medical emergency struck.

"We were having sex when his pain began. I'm Frank's wife, Janet. I knew it was bad, because he got sweatier than usual and what really got me worried is he didn't want to finish."

"Janet!" Mr. Thompson cries out.

"Thanks, that is very important information. Looking at your EKG and hearing your history, I have to inform you that you are having a little heart attack," I confide. I describe everybody's heart attacks as little even if they are not. It is only natural to get anxious after being told you had or are having a heart attack. The anxiety response that occurs with hearing the phrase, 'having a heart attack' can often trigger further catecholamine increase. Catecholamines that are most common: dopamine, epinephrine (adrenalin), and norepinephrine (noradrenalin). The surge of these in the bloodstream increases the stress response. Patients having a heart attack already have increased heart rate and blood pressure, so the balance of informing your patient in a calm manner is not only showing kindness, but it actually is providing good medical care. Terrible to say, but some could argue it might be better to hold off telling a patient they are having a heart attack. Then after treatment and resolution, you inform the patient completely and explain why you waited to inform them. I treat patients how I would like to be treated, but with an added layer of sugar coating. "Any prior cardiac history? Family members with heart disease? Smoking or other drug use, current or past? Problems with blood pressure? Sugar issues? cholesterol? etc." While I am asking more historical questions, I listen to my patient's heart and lungs. I access his pulses in all extremities and begin writing orders on a blue order sheet attached to Room 4's clipboard. My orders encompass lab tests and chest x-ray and include giving the patient aspirin and nitroglycerin under the tongue, known as sublingual. I ordered an IV dose of Lopressor, a beta-blocker that can lower both heart rate and blood pressure, lessening catecholamine response.

Unfortunately, my hospital's cardiac catheterization lab is not open on the weekends, and back then they only took patients weekdays 8AM to 5PM anyway. This doesn't mean my patient is without options. However, his best option will be delayed and I need to discuss a treatment called thrombolytic therapy. This is achieved by administering clot busting drugs in the IV and hoping to achieve lysis of the blockage in the particular coronary artery. If successful, then reperfusion occurs, which means blood flow is restored to the portion of heart muscle that had been cut off. After making sure my patient has no contraindications and going over the risks and benefits, I get Mr. Thompson's consent. I then order the thrombolytic medication. I also call the cardiologist at my nearest 24/7 cardiac catheterization lab and tell him about my patient. The doctor covering at the nearest hospital with the ability to perform the needed cardiac procedure gladly accepts Mr. Thompson. I give my patient and his wife the entire treatment strategy. The receiving heart doctor will often perform the catheterization procedure when my patient arrives at their institution, but time is precious. The hope is the thrombolytic opens the blockage and improves blood flow to the compromised heart muscle as quickly as possible. We continue cardiac monitoring throughout his time in the ED and often do serial EKGs.

Soon after the medication is given, my patient has a quick run of premature ventricular complexes (PVC's) indicating a likely reperfusion arrhythmia. It quickly resolves and my cardiac patient becomes pain free. In addition, his vital signs begin to normalize.

Blood Pressure: 139/85 Heart Rate: 90 Pulse Ox: 99%

As I am asking for a repeat EKG, Mr. Thompson asks, "Doc, what would have happened if I finished, you know, had an orgasm, would I have died?" He is looking at his wife as he asks me his question.

I grab a stool and sit down near the bedside so I am at his eye level. "It is possible, but there is only a slightly increased chance from finishing. What usually causes sudden death from a heart attack is when a non-perfusing cardiac arrhythmia occurs," I answer.

"See honey, you could have killed me. I told you your pussy would be the death of me," Mr. Thompson finishes while glaring at his wife. Javier, my tech, hands me the most recent EKG while I'm listening to Mr. Thompson inappropriately throwing blame at his wife. I look down at the EKG and see the ST elevations have lessened considerably but not completely.

"Hey now, Mr. Thompson, you are mistaken. Your wife or like you were alluding to, your wife's love area, didn't put your life in danger, but most likely because of her nether regions you are going to live." He was staring wide eyed at me as I now had his full attention. In addition, his wife's frown slowly turns into a smile. "Any strenuous activity most likely would have led to this heart attack. You could have been mowing the lawn, out for a run, or somewhere alone. You were lucky enough to be exerting not only with someone, but someone who knew you were in need of medical care. Thus, if not for your wife's willingness to offer herself for an exertional activity, you could still be sitting at home with a ticking time bomb in your chest. She defused it with possible little to no damage. I say you owe her some major thanks. Oh, don't forget a little praise to her love area wouldn't hurt," I finish with a slight chuckle. Both Mr. and Mrs. Thompson started laughing as she slowly stands up and hugs her husband. I can read in his face that he is a little ashamed that he blamed his wife's vagina because he was so fearful. While lying in bed, he hugs her back. Her hips are at his chest level so he wraps his arms around her waist. He gently places a kiss at her pubic region. Then with his arms still around her waist, he pulls back slightly with eyes focused at his wife's crotch area.

Mr. Thompson spoke to her crotch area, "Thank you pussy, I owe you my life." *I couldn't believe what I witnessed.* I stand up from the stool, thinking that's my cue to go check back in on the seizure boy. As I walk out of the room, *I start to think about the power of a woman's p.... A light-bulb suddenly goes off in my head. Why was Becca scratching around her private area?*

I race into Room 2. "Becca, why is your crotch itchy? Did your boyfriend use any special lotions?" I wait for a response as Nurse Sally tilts her head at me in a "Why would you ask such a thing?" manner?

Becca looks much more fatigued and is slumped a bit in her chair. "I'm feeling dizzy, things are blurry. Oh yeah, my pussy is all all numb, that's why it is really really itchy, it feels kinda funny, really weird like." Becca starts stuttering, almost acting like she is drunk and then closes her eyes.

I start shaking her gently and get her to focus. "Becca, what did you guys use?"

Her eyes open completely and she starts rambling and slowly mumbling her words. "Oh, Eric ordered some numbing stuff from a sexy catalog. He wanted to last long as possible. Got three tubes. He didn't eat it, just put it on his schlong and balls. I think he emptied a tube every time. He did it for me, he really really loves me. Cause it takes me a long long time to reach orgasm. I told him he put way too much on and kept reapplying anyway. He doesn't always listen to me, even though he loves me. I was feeling less and less, and so was taking me longer and longer to come and he didn't want to finish before me, but more cream wasn't helping me, only making him lots slower to orgasm. I'm startin to feelin funny," Becca finishes as she slumped back in her chair. *Holy shit!* He has lidocaine toxicity and she is now showing some signs and symptoms as well. lidocaine is a local anesthetic used commonly for simple procedures. Less common is its use at treating specific heart arrhythmias. The anesthetic form is injected subcutaneously but can come in a cream or jelly product.

"Sally, stop the Dilantin, I'm going to order Phenobarbital and more fluids. Get some soap and water and scrub his private area. Wait, I don't see a foley catheter? We need to put Becca in the bed next to him. Get one of the nurses to wash her privates and get IV fluids started and Ativan to bedside. I bet she starts seizing soon if we don't act. I think the Dilantin may have been making the toxicity worse." I was rambling because I was so excited I figured out the problem and could now focus on the solutions.

"Dr. A, I'm sorry I spaced on the foley," Sally apologizes.

"No problem, Sally. Stop the Dilantin and start the Phenobarb. *I wasn't sure, but I remembered Dilantin and Lidocaine had similar mechanisms of action.* My selection of Dilantin in this toxicity case may have exacerbated the Lidocaine's effects. The Phenobarb, a barbiturate, is better for drug poisoning induced seizures. It turned out that Eric's entire crotch was caked in a thin, clear Lidocaine jelly residue. My pushing to get to CT and then do the LP caused Sally to forget to place the catheter in his penis. She would have noticed the thick residue all over his private area. I can't throw all the blame at Sally. In all honesty, I should have stripped the patient completely naked. Once naked, I should have done a more thorough physical exam. With my cursory examination, I did not discover the material on his privates. I don't routinely grope patient's testicles and penises unless that is the location of their chief complaint. Becca, the girlfriend, wasn't helpful. In her defense, she was suffering ill effects from the Lidocaine as well. Doctors often come up with justification for our misses or delays, as in this case. Removing the source of toxicity is paramount. Unfortunately, we were delayed, or rather I missed it. Better late than never. Once we knew the source, I also had one of my nurses call poison control and run our case by them to get any additional recommendations they might have. They were surprised the benzodiazepines didn't work and agreed that the Phenobarb was the correct selection. Will his stable blood pressure and no cardiac rhythm abnormalities, poison control advised against giving the Lidocaine antidote of lipid emulsion, which I have only seen used once in my career. Eric's seizures never recurred once the Phenobarb started infusing and Dilantin was pulled. At that point in my career, Eric and his numb penis was the first Lidocaine toxicity patient I had ever encountered. Currently 5% Lidocaine cream can be purchased without prescription. My seizure patient was able to obtain prescription strength without a script. Worse than that, he over applied big time.

Becca never had a seizure and made a complete recovery. She was discharged about ten hours later. She spent the night in one of our observation rooms. Eric wasn't as lucky. He spent the next two days in the Intensive Care Unit (ICU). I recall Eric's lab did show an elevation of Creatine Kinase (CK), showing an increased level of muscle damage from the seizures. This led to a mild case of Rhabdomyolysis (Rhabdo for short). Rhabdo is when damage to muscle tissue causes protein and electrolytes to enter the bloodstream, causing harm to various organs, commonly kidneys and sometimes the heart. He also showed some delayed cognitive findings that were resolved before he went home. The day after the bloody full moon shift I looked up the product he used and found that he took almost 300 times the recommended application.

These two cases dealt with life threatening sexual encounters from which everyone can learn. Number one, make sure to treat your partner's privates with kindness and respect, as they may someday save your life. Secondly, when it comes to your own privates, don't act like a dumb ass or you may end up with something more serious than numb nuts.

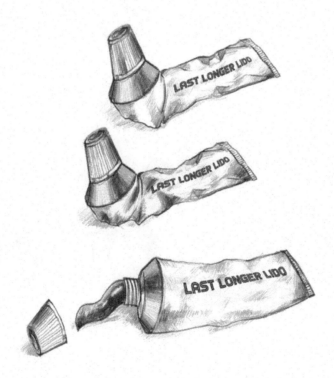

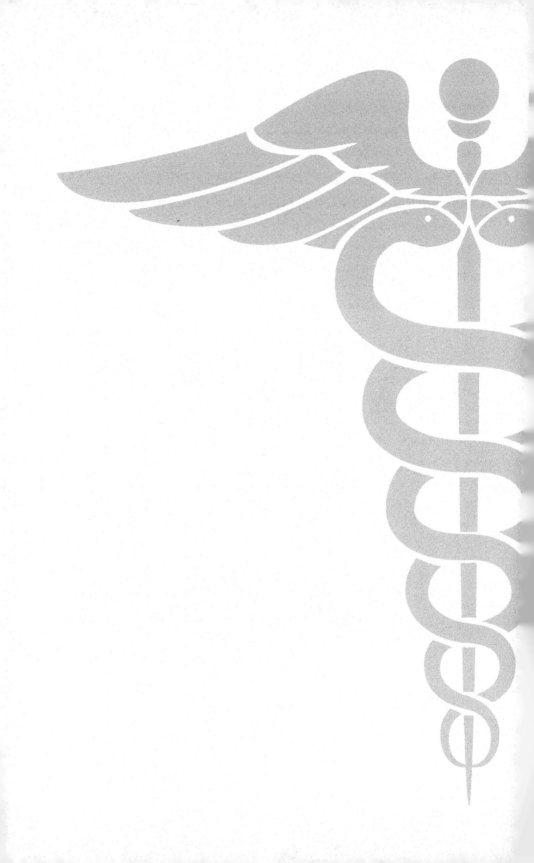

CHAPTER 3

Emergency Department
Staff 9 p.m.

I'd be remiss if I did not give you a description of the emergency department staff. EDs, like any working environment, depend on the employees who staff them. Each new shift, I assess the scheduled nurses on that particular day. Today I was blessed with many who play for the A team. Sally and Betty have a few hours to go on their 12-hour shift, but two nurses, Judy and Melody recently arrived. Melody is the rookie and replacing another newbie nurse. The department runs better when you split up the less experienced nurses to different shifts. Some departments have many who could be A team members. Most places of business have their share of poor performers. When a shift is covered by all the rotten apples, well it sucks. Usually the quality, or lack of, in a shift's nurses determines how smoothly my particular work day will be. Of course, the patients and their problems may have some say to how my day goes. In addition to my nurses, in this particular emergency department, paramedics work side by side with them. Usually, local EMS are not directly employed by hospitals, but by outside institutions. The ambulances and crews are often headquartered separately from the hospitals. The hospital I worked at right out of residency was the exception. There, paramedics were employed by the hospital and their ambulance station was connected to the hospital parking lot. Our hospital did a good job balancing the two varying disciplines. Paramedics not only have to be quick movers and thinkers, but independent. When they are in the field, they have to make decisions and act accordingly and are not depending on doctors instruction or supervision. Likewise, emergency nurses self-select working in the ED because they happen to be quick thinkers and movers. However, they are trained to be dependent on doctors and taught to suppress their independent inclinations. Both have overlapping skills and interest in treating the variety of patients who present to the ED. As it so happened, half of my paramedics were also registered nurses (RNs) who pulled shifts as both medic or nurse at different times. Additional staff include the clerks or secretaries that field calls, put in orders, and function as central command of an emergency department (tonight Cindy has that role). We have emergency technicians (techs) who often have a practical nurse degree (LPN) and assist with EKGs, splinting, transporting, cleaning, and lifting patients (Javier today). They basically perform everything and anything you could think of that requires extra hands. Other department workers often spend a lot of time doing their job in the ED, but belong to other hospital areas such as respiratory technicians, phlebotomists, social workers, and radiology personnel. The radiology technicians include an ultrasound tech and sometimes both a CT and separate plain X-ray tech. Tonight, Jane is doing both CT and plain imaging. Depending on the hospital and ED's current patients, security and police personnel can be fixtures as well.

Two of today's paramedics, Kyle and Jason, walk into the ED looking fresh and rested. Their twelve-hour shift started at 7:00 p.m. Both are under thirty years old, with people sometimes confusing Jason for me with his similar tall, skinny build, and brown hair. On the other extreme is Kyle, who has a stocky, very muscular build, and his blond hair in a mullet style. Another benefit of in-house paramedics is they often can provide much needed muscle when called upon. I'm not weak, but most of the female paramedics are nearly as strong as I and most of the male medics could squash me like a bug. I very much like the thought of extra muscle a quick yell away. The only thing better is an armed police officer hanging out in the ED. All hospitals have security personnel, but that doesn't mean they can handle unruly patients. The problem is half of hospital security seems to be made up of pretty women less than 100 lbs. It seems somebody hired them to soothe the savage beast. That rarely works for the hostile ER animal. The other half are large, scary dudes at least six foot five and 300lbs. These guys are usually teddy bears. The problem is that the large teddy bears have never had a single fight in their entire life. No one in their right mind would ever want to fight them. They are too scary looking. So, of course, when a violent patient starts swinging at staff, who do you call? The best process is to inform the in-house paramedics and give a ring to the police as back up. The reality is the medics like action and they will often act before being told. Hell, that is why they became paramedics in the first place. Nurses by nature are helpers. A helper's first thought is not to tackle or subdue, but assist a person in need. Unfortunately, we get patients who sometimes need a six-foot 2 x 4 board to the head. Ok, that's poor ED humor. But sedation and a jail cell is what a particularly troublesome patient may really need. Thankfully, we have excellent medication that can create sleepy-time without leaving a mark on the skull or other permanent damage. My job is not only to fix broken bones, but to prevent any of my staff or the patient from obtaining new broken body parts. At least while they're in my ER.

Jason gets my attention, then informs me that police have brought in a new patient. Usually if police don't call paramedics at the scene, then rarely is the case a true medical emergency. Police bring patients to the ED for multiple reasons. The majority are for medical clearance for jail or simple blood draws for suspected driving under the influence. The medical clearance cases are often for suicidal or other psychiatric issues. With real injuries or actual suicidal attempts, the medics are called and police usually defer transport to the medical providers. That is unless there is a high concern for violence from the patient. "Doc, the new dude got tased 6 times. That's before he kicked out the squad car's back window. They say he downed a bunch of MDMA as they were chasing him down. The officers are pissed big time. Kyle and I are going out to take a quick picture of their car," Jason informed me as I heard some yelling coming from Room 5.

MDMA stands for 3,4 Methylenedioxy-Methamphetamine. It is a synthetic stimulant/psychedelic often called Ecstasy or Molly. Its properties vary from Meth, another amphetamine often termed Ice or Speed. MDMA is often taken orally in pill or powder form whereas Meth is often inhaled or injected. MDMA doesn't have as many devastating long-term effects as Meth, but it does have some. Over time, cognitive damage resulting in memory and emotional dysfunction can result. Meth's long-term problems can affect every bodily system from tooth decay to causing some users to become cardiac cripples before they even are twenty years old. Short term because Meth's route of use is smoking it, can lead to respiratory issues. In addition, injecting it can lead to skin or other infections. In my experience, all Meth contains additional toxic substances. MDMA will often contain Fentanyl or other unknown component additions. Local communities don't have Walter White making their drugs.

Walking quickly toward the noise, I see Nurse Judy's attempt to get vitals rebuffed. The patient is lying mostly supine, with his right wrist handcuffed to the bed. An officer is at the head of the bed, pinning the patient's shoulders. A middle-aged dude wearing grungy clothes who won't stop moving is my next patient. His long, matted brown hair is stuck to a thin coat of blood that covers most of his face. Judy was unsuccessfully trying to place the blood pressure cuff on the man's left arm. He was kicking his legs and flailing his left arm. "Let's put him in four-point leather restraints. We can do IM (intramuscular) Haldol (an antipsychotic medication). Then we can get an IV and medicate more as needed," I order.

"Yes!" Kyle yips as he jumps on top of the flailing patient's legs. Kyle had popped out of nowhere. He and Jason were lightning quick, taking pictures of the kicked out back window. Kyle doesn't like missing any action. Jason quickly brought over the leather restraints. To the casual observer, the restraints definitely look medieval. That's even before we attach them. The four separate thick cowhide leather straps have ends that have metal locking mechanisms that clang when carried. A rat couldn't chew through these in under a year. We cinch his two wrists and two ankles, then attach the other ends to the bed railings. The flailing is nullified, even before the IM medication. Soon after we snug the restraints tight, he stops fighting. We didn't even need to administer any medication.

I look over at the oldest of the two police officers. "What's the story?"

The officer is not happy, but looking down at his lawbreaker now shackled lightens his mood. "Well Doc, this piece of trash was selling Ecstasy outside the school. We got a tip from one of the prom chaperones. When we pulled up, he bolted. We saw him stuff his mouth while running. There were no drugs on his person. This isn't his first rodeo. He was out of breath when we threw him in the back of the squad car. Heading to the station he started flipping out. The piece of shit kicked out our back window and cut his face up trying to crawl out. Don't worry, we were stopped when he tumbled out. Hell, if he wasn't bleeding we wouldn't even have brought him in."

"Thanks, officer. Judy, please clean up his face and give Valium if he starts acting up again."

One, if not the, most overlooked variables that separate EDs around the country is police assistance. Throughout my twenty-five years in emergency medicine, I have been licensed and worked in six states. As I am sure you know, our laws across this great land vary considerably. What might be of insight is that law enforcement's legal power affects the emergency physician's job greatly. Depending on what state the hospital is in and sometimes the patient's legal residency can determine the type of care one gets. Not to fear, we emergency health care providers evaluate every single patient who comes in the door. Or we are legally required to, anyway. Specifically, we are federally mandated by law to perform an exam. We term this a "medical screening exam," and it includes more than taking vitals in triage. However, people think that we are legally required to treat them. We are not! Rending treatment is not mandated, unless we deem that there might be a problem that could lead to morbidity or mortality, without said treatment. After we examine a patient and determine no medical emergency exists, we can stop right there. Sometimes we need a test or two to determine if an emergent medical problem exists. Often we can determine the level of need with a quick history and physical exam and then our legal responsibility can end.

The legal power of law enforcement is an entirely different matter. Responsibility varies from state to state. Some states defer to the ED physician, while other states give the police officer the final say. Yes, even pertaining to medical decisions. Example: In one case, police brought a 20-year-old male to the ED, who told his ex-girlfriend he planned to kill himself. They want a medical clearance from me and then they would take him to the psychiatric hospital for 48-hour hold. I review his vitals, do a quick physical, and sign off. He is clear, medically. The next patient is also a 20-year-old male, brought in by police officers, but he lives across the border in a different state. They say the patient voiced suicidal thoughts to neighbors but not to them or anybody else. I (or if I decide to defer to my psychiatrist on call) will be the judge of whether he needs hospitalization or not. I decided, usually after getting my psychiatrist's opinion, he isn't suicidal and he goes home. So, depending on where the patient resides and sometimes where the event occurred determines who is responsible for their health care decisions. Not that big of a deal you say. Well, the first 20-year-old male never told his ex he wanted to kill himself. She was pissed that he broke it off with her and she called the police and lied to them. She knew that they might send the boy to a psychiatric hospital just on her word. That is exactly what occurred. I told the police my suspicion about her making up the story. The officer said the kid will only be hospitalized for the weekend or until the psychiatrist sees him. Well, that really sucked for him and frustrated me.

This is one small example. The concern is the inconsistency regarding who has legal responsibility. Our MDMA ingesting patient would be sitting in a padded jail cell in one state even with injuries, versus being dumped in my ED for the entire night in a different state, injury free. In fact, sometimes a possible medical injury can be a get-out-of-jail-free card. They drop an injured criminal at the ER and the police officers hit the road. Cops don't want to wait, and if the patient didn't murder anybody or anybody important, they vamoose. The patient gets treated and walks out the door a free man. Slight exaggeration, but you'd be surprised who walks away without any consequences. Lots of variability exists between state laws that give law enforcement different protection. I'm not going to take sides or debate for more or less legal power for our law enforcement. It is a double-edged sword. I don't want 100% responsibility every time, but I also don't want zero control ever.

Here is an interesting, but very sad case. A young new mom of twins was brought in by police for insomnia. The day before, social services went to the house and took custody of the two ten-day-old twins. The mother had been cleaning the kitchen table for the past four days. This was non-stop, 24-hours-a-day cleaning, one particular table, and doing nothing else. Family took over infant care and gave the new mom food and water. They forced food and drink down her while she continued to scrub the table. She would defecate and urinate while standing, not stopping her cleaning. The mom did not sleep, but continued to wash and wipe the table hour after hour, never stopping. The police officer brought her in and said that she wasn't suicidal, so he would not be taking her to the psychiatric hospital for care. The officer wanted me to give her medication and he would drive her home. In that particular state, I did not have the power to override his decision. This woman clearly needed hospitalization in a psychiatric facility. The problem was she said "no" when the officer asked if she was suicidal. She was not in her right mind to answer that question and I needed to persuade him to change his mind. This tragic patient had postpartum psychosis. This is an extremely terrible problem that we hear in appalling news reports when new mothers kill their babies and/or children. I am very persuasive, but after an hour, I still had to get my psychiatrist to assist in changing the officer's mind. This situation was obvious, or so I thought, but in the more subtle cases, patients can fall through the cracks. We can have too much power, or not enough. I include these cases to highlight some unique challenges that occur in emergency departments across this great country.

Nurse Judy soon had the restrained patient's face clean and hair nicely pulled back. Judy is one of my "nurse pluggers"—kind of like a utility player on a baseball team. She fills whatever role is needed. If I have a patient who only requires a compassionate ear or kind voice, Judy can fill that need. If there is a serious life and death issue where we have to act quickly, Judy can handle that as well. If I need no judgment but diligent action, like efficient cleaning of my MDMA soon-to-be a jailbird patient, Judy's reliable. Judy also has a quiet contentment that enables her to be calm when chaos builds. Part of that stems from having her new girlfriend working at the hospital—Jane, our CT technician. Judy also puts Jane in a happy mood when Jane enters the ED to grab a patient for the CAT scanner.

As a result of Judy's diligence, our patient was all cleaned up and prepared for me to assess the extent of the facial damage. There was a large hematoma above his left eye that gravity would shift downwards, causing that eye to be swollen shut by morning. He also had about six or seven superficial facial lacerations. These would come together well with our adhesive or super glue for skin. "Hey Doc, are you going to make our patient all pretty so the other inmates will get turned on when we bring him to jail?" the police officer chides. He is still upset about their squad car's back window being kicked out. He wants to tease the patient because there wasn't much else he could do to get even, other than the multiple tasing they already administered. The patient starts fighting the restraints and growled back at the officer.

"Don't get him riled up before I glue those cuts. Come on man!" I like to do a good job on my lacerations, and a moving target doesn't help. As I position myself over his face armed with my small adhesive tube, I notice how huge his eyelashes are, especially his upper lid lashes. I'm about to remark on them, but figure the officers will totally rip into his feminine features. The problem is, one of the lacerations is a half inch below his right eye. It is just in range of his freakishly long eyelashes. Lacerations near the eyes is one of the locations where we substitute sutures (stitches). Even on small wounds that will do better with adhesive, we don't want to take a chance to glue someone's eye shut for a week. I finish closing six wounds, leaving the one near his eye for last. I look at the patient and tell him, "I need to use sutures for your last cut because it is too close to your eye. Or I can let it heal on its own and you'll probably have a little bigger scar."

"No! I don't want a scar. Why can't you use the glue?" the patient blurts out. I was shocked at how coherent he was and realize this guy was acting out more from him being a pain in the ass than any drug effects.

"Well, I don't want your eyelashes hitting the glue. Your eye will be closed shut for at least four to five days."

"He does have such pretty eyelashes, Doc. The guys in jail might think he is a girl," the officer couldn't resist saying. Mr. Eyelashes started fuming and growled louder than last time.

I look back at the officer, "Argh, what did I say?" I then turn my attention to my restrained patient. "Ok, I'll use the glue if you want, but I'll hold your eye open for at least one minute or that eyelash will touch the glue."

"Ok, ok! Just get it done," my lovely patient answers. With my left hand, I held Mr. Window-kicker's eyelashes back and brought my right hand with the adhesive tube toward the wound. Sometimes the glue comes out faster than anticipated, but I had recently done a number of cuts and knew how much pressure to apply to get the perfect amount needed. I gently squeezed the tube and closed the wound with near perfect precision. Now I only need to hold the eye open for 60 seconds. The glue dries quickly.

Suddenly, the officer chimes in one more time. "Oh boy, Doc, he's even prettier than before." The patient had enough and jerks his head toward the officer. My finger loses contact with his eyelid. The fuming patient blinks his eyes, and this results in his huge upper eyelashes coming down and contacting the glue. The connection of glue and eyelashes instantly bond. The glue's strong effect caused slight discomfort from the attracting forces, causing the patient to close his eyes even tighter. This makes even more eyelashes ensnare in the glue, sealing his eye completely. It would now be shut tight for days. The officers roar with laughter. The patient goes ballistic. I look at his good left eye and realize that chances are that by morning all the blood from that hematoma would drain down, resulting in his left eyelid to swell. This would leave him unable to see out of either eye.

"Judy, please put an ice pack on his left eyebrow." I request.

A few minutes later, the police officers get called away. They are needed for a large unplanned raid of some sort. They need to leave soon, with or without cyclops. "You guys can have him. I'm done. Have him keep ice on his left eyebrow," I instruct.

The patient yells, "I don't need the fuckin ice, get it off."

The two officers look at each other and I could tell they had figured why I had been adamant about applying ice. I see understanding behind their devious eyes. They have no intention of offering any more ice. We take off the restraints and they reapply the handcuffs. Before the officers escort the patient out the door, they stop by my desk, "Doc, you don't know how much we appreciated that. Thanks!" To this day I think they thought I did it on purpose. That wasn't the case, but at least it happened to somebody that kind of deserved it.

"Doc, I heard you glued that dude's eye shut. Damn! I would have loved seeing that. Well, there is one thing that I'd like to see more than almost anything else. You know what that is, right, Doc? Maybe I'll get to take care of Batman's girlfriend later tonight," Kyle remarks. Jason, his partner for the entire night, shook his head in response. Kyle was the rookie medic to Jason's veteran status. Kyle had high energy, full of vim and vigor. Jason wasn't much older, but had been a medic right out of high school. Jason was one of the few medics who I trusted as much as the paramedics who were also RNs. Jason studied medicine and was always eager to learn about even the boring medical happenings in the ED. Kyle was a different case entirely. He was in it for the adrenaline rush. Trauma cases, cardiac arrest, anybody dying or close to it, Kyle was right on hand. The run of the mill, some would say boring patients, Kyle was in the back doing paperwork. "Doc, I heard about some of the crazy sex patients you already had tonight. Oh man, I knew tonight would be awesome with that killer blood moon. It was turning a bloody brown color when I drove in a few minutes ago. Once that sun is completely gone, mayhem will ensue. I can't wait. So, you think Batman is having sex right now?" Kyle asks me.

Kyle was obsessed with one particular paramedic urban legend. The story possibly could be true, but I had only heard paramedics talk about it and never saw it in a medical journal or other reputable source. Some say it was Halloween, others say it was simply a night with a full moon. Two paramedics get a simple call about a bleeding unconscious man and a woman yelling. The police had called for a paramedic standby. What that entails is having the paramedics on scene but awaiting police to access and secure the area before calling in the medical personnel. The setting was an apartment complex on the second floor. A neighbor heard a woman yelling and dialed 911. The police arrived and heard a frantic woman screaming her brains out. She was so hysterical they couldn't determine exactly what was going on. She kept yelling, "His head's bleeding and he isn't moving. I don't know if he's breathing. Help! Help!" The police yelled for her to open the door. Her response was, "I'm tied up, get in here. Help! Help!"

When the medics heard her say his head was bleeding and he wasn't moving, they ran up the stairs and begged the police to break the door down immediately. The police were going to do that, but supposedly this apartment complex was a local drug haven. They wanted to be careful and didn't want to rush into an ambush and get shot. The paramedics consisted of an older veteran past his prime but still fit and fast acting. The other was a rookie, ready to save every patient or die trying. The paramedics, so the story goes, pushed the police aside and kicked down the door. The two medics ran to the back room where the screaming was coming from, disregarding the police instructing them to wait. Both medics arrived simultaneously. The veteran medic accessed the scene quickly. A beautiful blond thirty something woman was lying in bed totally naked. She was spread eagle with ankles tied to both lower corner bedposts and wrists to the upper posts. A naked man wearing only a Batman cowl and cape was lying on the ground with blood coming from his head. A ceiling fan spinning rapidly was directly over the bed. The veteran paramedic knew immediately what had transpired. The man had tied up his woman and proceeded to climb the end of the bed. He must have leapt too high and hit his head on the fan, knocking himself out. Before the police arrived the veteran medic turned to the rookie, pointed at the woman, and said, "I'll take care of her! You save Batman!"

Kyle loved that story. The idea of a beautiful naked woman and a bleeding, unconscious patient was his dream ambulance run. "Kyle, I bet we will have plenty of walk-ins who will provide excitement all night long. Don't wish for more, please," I beg.

"Welcome to my world, Doc. Let us know where you need us," Jason adds. Jason's experience and calming manner were vital to keep Kyle from getting too rambunctious. I admittedly was like Kyle during my residency years. I wanted to see everything and get my hands dirty. I couldn't get enough blood and guts, or patients with life and death on the line. You name it, I wanted to see and treat it all. As the young inexperienced resident, I wanted mayhem and chaos not for the thrill, but for the exposure aspect. I figured the more experiences with every imaginable and unimaginable patient the better physician I'd be. Most people don't realize what leads to the adrenalin rush. Is the fact of having someone's life is in your hands? Trying to solve an unsolvable problem? The scream of a suffering patient's voice? For me, as a physician, the major adrenalin factor was from not knowing what the hell I was doing. I wanted to achieve mastery of having no adrenalin rush during the most chaotic times. A busy emergency department can be like a tornado of chaos. I wanted mastery of that chaos. Knowledge and thus confidence of what to do in every situation that is presented in my ED was my ultimate goal. Simply put, I wanted to be like a Shaolin monk of the ED. I wanted supreme knowledge and experience in all situations. If I was able to achieve that mastery, then I could control my adrenalin release. The hope was that in crazier and highly stressful cases, my control would enable me to be calmer and approach a Zen like state. I wanted calmness in mind and body, but roadrunner fast inside my brain. Similar to the appearance of a graceful swan, looking calm and controlled above the water but below the surface frantic legs churning or in my case brain sorting diagnostic and treatment plans. Over the years, my mastery of adrenalin has improved considerably. However good my speed of problem solving and Zen-like might appear, I still have yet to achieve a complete emotional controlled level. At times when chaos is raining down in the ED and patients, nurses, ancillary staff are all moving around like chickens with their heads cut off, I attempt to calmly hold them all together. With me leading my team into each medical emergency battle, we will endeavor to bring each of our patients the quickest and safest victory possible.

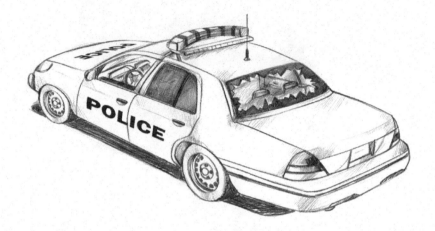

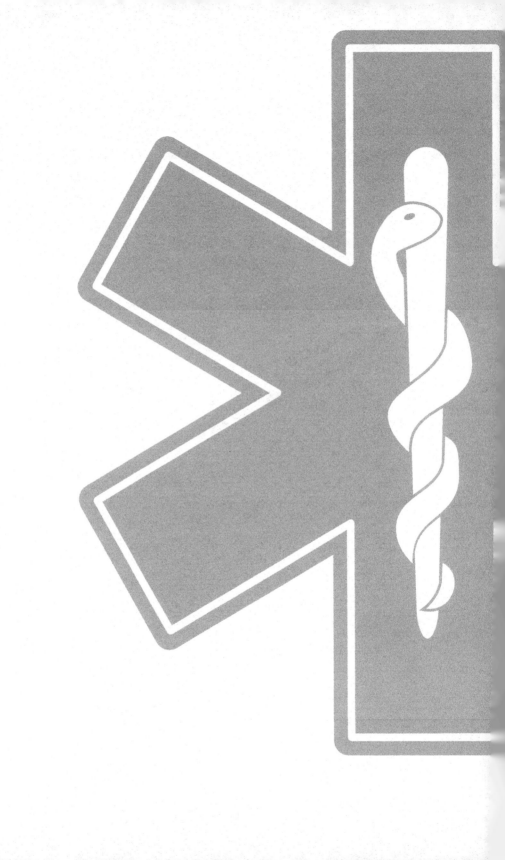

CHAPTER 4

That doesn't look right 9:19 p.m.

The human body is miraculous and incredibly resilient, but sometimes it mysteriously over reacts. Those mysterious reactions can be devastating. Some bodies develop autoimmune disorders like Rheumatoid arthritis (RA) or Multiple Sclerosis (MS) among them. Even more deadly than an autoimmune disease is the cancer cell that our own body produces and proliferates into a large life-threatening problem. This book is about emergency medicine which are acute or sudden problems. An acute over reaction can be seen with a simple allergic response, such as a swollen arm from an insect bite or poison ivy contact. When the allergy affects the entire body, we use the term "systemic," referring to an entire system. This can lead to an anaphylactic reaction. Anaphylaxis is a severe, life-threatening allergic reaction. Medically speaking, it occurs when the body has an acute allergic reaction to an antigen (bee sting, nut, drug) to which the body has become hypersensitive. Why does someone's body over react to eating a nut, swallowing a particular drug, or a simple bee sting? I'm not going to answer that. What I am going to share is the funniest EMS call of my career. `

Medics called in a severe anaphylaxis patient. I know, there is nothing funny about a life- threatening presentation. Well, maybe there is? CC: Left ear pain 6-year-old male.

I am pleasantly surprised looking down on my next chart. Happily, I walk toward the ear patient's room and quickly try to forget about my earlier patients. I have already seen my share of unique encounters in the first three hours of the shift. If the rest of my shift brings boring, simple, and easy patient problems, I'll not complain. After seeing the smiling talkative little boy with the swollen right ear drum, I walk back to my desk. I quickly write out a prescription for the antibiotic Amoxicillin, and print out ear infection instructions.

BEEP! BEEP! BEEP! The EMS radio blares. *Wow, my eardrums are going to be as swollen as my recent little patient's if we can't get that damn radio volume figured out.* The high volume continues over the radio as the dispatcher informs paramedics of their next call: "WE HAVE 40-YEAR-OLD WOMAN HAVING SEVERE ALLERGIC REACTION AFTER ELEPHANT TRUNK PENETRATED VAGINA! REPEAT WOMAN HAVING SEVERE ALLERGIC REACTION ON 1ST AND GRAND, APARTMENT 101!" I stop a few feet from handing a prescription to the mom of my young ear infection patient. My brain is trying to register the EMS call. *Did they say an elephant penetrated a vagina?*

"Hells yeah!" Kyle whoops and tells Jason to meet him out front. He'll sprint to the ambulance, pull it around front, then grab Jason at the edge of the hospital parking lot. *At least somebody is excited for tonight's unending mayhem.*

I look down at the young six-year-old boy and wonder if he was listening to the paramedic radio call. My question is answered as I hear the six-year-old boy ask his mom, "Mommy are they going to bring the severely reacting lady with the elephant vagina here?" Smiling, I hand his mom the script and discharge instructions. The mother is left speechless, her eyes pleading for the nearest exit.

Emergency departments have EMS radios to communicate with their paramedics in the field. Some departments, like ours, listen to the dispatcher calls because of our in-house paramedics. Accuracy on the dispatch calls is often questionable. The 911 operator is often receiving verbal information from a frantic patient or family member. I don't get worked up until the paramedics arrive on the scene and give us their interpretation of the complaint and situation. A dispatch example that was completely inaccurate happened only a week before this shift. The dispatcher told the paramedics a pregnant woman was in severe labor, delivering a goat. It turned out our local petting zoo owner was assisting her goat's birth when her own water broke and the husband dialed 911 in his over emotional reaction. So, I always chill out until I hear what the paramedics have to say. I trust their eyes more than a random, often frantic person. *We'll know the real story soon enough as the address for the allergic reaction patient is only five minutes aways. Also, I was pretty sure the local petting zoo didn't have any elephants.*

After the loud EMS call, I did look around the department and noticed every nurse, Cindy the clerk, and Javier the tech wearing big smiles and chuckling about what they heard. "Don't get too excited, guys. Let's wait until the medics give us their report before we get our butts in a knot," I laugh.

Ten minutes later my sphincter tightens. BEEP! BEEP! BEEP! "MEDIC 1 REPORT, 5 MINUTES OUT WITH 40, REPEAT 40-YEAR-OLD WOMAN IN ANAPHYLAXIS AFTER ELEPHANT TRUNK PENETRATED..."

Before the medic could finish, a frantic, hyperventilating woman's voice screams, "MY PUSSY, MY PUSSY, MY PUSSY!"

The medic tries to continue, "MEDIC 1 REPEATING, 40-YEAR-OLD WOMAN 5 MINUTES OUT WITH ANAPHYLACTIC REACTION AFTER ELEPHANT TRUNK

PENETRATED HER…"

"MY PUSSY, MY PUSSY, MY PUSSY," the woman screams again.

"ARRGGHH!!! MEDIC 1 BE THERE SOON, UNABLE TO GET BP, ATTEMPTING IV, OU!, MY PU…" Radio cut out.

I grab the EMS radio microphone. Pressing down on the intercom, "ER COPIES, MEDIC 1, SEE YOU IN 5, ER OUT!" I turn around with a big grin on my face, looking to make eye contact with my staff. "It's real. *Maybe?* Let's prep Trauma room 3. Grab fluids, Epinephrine, Solu-Medrol (IV steroid), IV Benadryl (antihistamine), and IV Valium (a benzodiaze-pine). We'll assess what's really going on before we push any medicines." My guess was that the patient was having an allergic reaction and asso-ciated anxiety response causing her hyperventilation. I had a good guess where the reaction was taking place, but with her screaming so loud I had my doubts against her experiencing a true anaphylactic reaction.

The ambulance pulls up and before the bay doors open we all hear "MY PUSSY, MY PUSSY, MY PUSSY!" The doors part and paramedics Jason and Kyle are pushing the gurney into the ED. Kyle no longer looks as excited as when he exited the ED 20 minutes ago. I point to Room 3 and follow as they wheel in a semi-attractive, brunette hair shooting in all directions, 40-something patient.

"Doc, we got the IV as we pulled up, so we haven't given any medi-cation yet," Paramedic Kyle informs me. In seconds, Betty and Melody are hooking the patient up to the monitor and flushing the medic's IV (a way to access or clear IV, often with a syringe filled with saline fluid or heparin, a blood thinner medicine). I look at the patient. She is breathing very fast, cheeks are flushed. She is wearing a blue t-shirt and a blanket is covering her from the waist down. I grab her wrist and feel a strong, fast pulse. I'm getting reassured that I'm not dealing with an anaphylactic reaction. I look at the monitor: Blood Pressure: 190/95 Pulse Ox: 99%

A life-threatening anaphylactic situation typically arises from two scenarios: either severe hypotension, which is life threatening low blood pressure, or airway obstruction due to swelling. Occasionally, both may occur simultaneously, which is really scary. Symptoms are often feeling lightheaded, difficulty breathing, increased heart rate, anxiety, clammy skin, confusion, and possible loss of consciousness. This patient did have some of the aforementioned mentioned symptoms. However, her blood pressure reassured me and there was no issue with her airway. She is having a hyperventilation syndrome and probably a localized allergic reaction. "Hello, I am Dr. Adams, Mrs...."

"MY PUSSY, MY PUSSY, MY PUSSY," she answers me.

I look over at Betty. "Hold all meds except give the Valium, now!" Betty acknowledges me with her eyes and mouths a "Thank you" response. One minute after the Valium was pushed into her IV with a bag of Normal Saline (NS) running, the patient's breathing slows and her next, "My Pussy, My Pussy, My Pussy" volume only projects into the hall, not throughout the entire ED. I am able to look into the back of her throat and do not appreciate any gross swelling or redness. Her exposed skin also seems clear of any rashes or redness. With how loud she was yelling about her private area, I was sure she didn't have any airway problems. I need to look at her private area as that is definitely the patient's main concern. Looking around the room, I notice way more people than I need present when I access a patient's private area. Both paramedics, Kyle, and Jason, are still at bedside. The majority of the time they bolt as soon as they are done moving the patient from the gurney to bed. I see a phlebotomist and x-ray tech in the corner of the room. What the hell, a janitor is standing at the door entrance peeking in. "Ok, everybody out except Betty and Melody," I instruct. *I understand people's curiosity and everybody in the entire ED knows what I am about to be looking at, but come on man.*

After all nonessential hospital employees vacate, I get Melody's attention and point to the stirrups at the end of bed. Melody pulls both stirrups out and then gently lifts the patient's legs, resting her feet on each stirrup footpad. My patient is now spread eagle and still covered in her large thick greenish blanket. I reach down grabbing, the blanket about to expose her...

"Honey, My Pussy! My Pussy! My Pussy!" I look at my patient, and see her eyes are staring at the doorway. Following their path reveals an average-built, middle-aged man who looks surprisingly disheveled while wearing a fancy dress shirt and slacks. His shirt is untucked and his hair is a chaotic mess. He is carrying a large brown paper bag. The bag is extended from his chest like the contents have radioactive material inside. His eyes look red and puffy like he has been sobbing, or had way too much to drink. *Probably both.*

"Is the elephant inside?" Betty asks, eyeing the bag like a little girl receiving a birthday present. Before he can answer, Betty snatches the bag and places it on the counter near the sink.

"What about my pussy?" My patient finally speaks her first complete sentence and stops after saying pussy only once. *Progress.*

"We can look in the bag after we see, um, under the blanket." I fumble my words. I'm thinking this is really interesting but also might be nasty and visually scarring. I pause, then look around the room, meeting everybody's eyes to make sure everybody is ready for the big reveal. Betty and

Melody look way too excited. The husband is close to wimping out as his hands are practically covering his eyes. The patient's eyes are closed shut. I hold my breath and pull off the blanket. Betty and Melody move into the visual range of the patient's crotch area. The husband spreads his fingers apart so his vision is no longer obstructed and cries out, "My wife's poor pussy, poor pussy, poor pussy!" Tears start flowing from his eyes. I'm betting he wished he kept his eyes covered for the unveiling. I look down and realize that this visual will leave a scar on any man's libido, especially if that man was the cause for this. Her poor vagina was so grotesquely swollen and misshapen it no longer resembled human tissue. Her labia looked like two beefy red deflated footballs being pushed apart by inner vaginal tissue that was protruding outwards. The vaginal tissue reminded me of the alien from the original Alien movie bursting out of the stomach, but in this case her vagina. I decided to give it a nickname, like "Vagalien" (pronounced vahj-alien). When a traumatic or scary visual transcends reality, humor can help one cope. In addition, like many medical professionals, I always like to have a handy sensational patient story to share during a night out with friends. Great drinking stories need a monster and Vagalien sounds great for a scary monster name. *Sounds terrible, but one has to get their entertainment somewhere.*

Women can develop vaginal, uterine, or rectal prolapse. This occurs when pelvic muscles and or ligaments weaken. This can result in a protrusion of said anatomy. This Vagalien was different because technically nothing prolapsed but it still protruded. The magnitude of the swollen tissue made it look as if the anatomy had moved. In reality, it was actually extremely distorted giving it an alien appearance. "Melody, give Benadryl, Solu-Medrol, and get a bunch of ice packs," I gently order. I stare at the vaginal tissue. *If I get too close it will jump out and bite me. I need to tread lightly and not make this tissue mad at me.*

All of a sudden, the patient grabs my hand making me jump. "Doctor, how bad is my pussy? It feels so bad, I can't look!" I want to reassure her, but it really looks bad. I have a tendency to inform my patients with a straight answer, to the point where I am often accused of being too blunt. *This will be hard to sugarcoat.*

"It's not life threatening," I answer. *But if your husband stares too long at this, your sex life is dead.* "The nurse is giving you medicine that will help with the swelling. She is going to apply ice and I'll add some IV morphine for the pain so you can tolerate the discomfort. We can give you more Valium," I finish. *God, I hope that was enough reassurance.* My patient has severe contact dermatitis. The closest usual comparison would be a poison ivy reaction from the deepest depths of hell isolated to her poor vagina and labia.

"Hey Doc, we should look at the elephant," Betty chimes in, wanting to examine the second surprise gift. I turn to the brown paper bag sitting on the counter. Thankfully, the counter is located at the head of the bed, so my patient is facing away from the brown bag. I don't know if examining the bag's contents will help me shake the beefy red vaginal image, or solidify that picture. I take a few steps toward the bag. *Well at least I'm walking away from the Vagalien.* I slowly uncurl the crinkled top portion and open the bag. Peering in, I see a gray painted ceramic elephant the size of an average chihuahua. I pull it out. *Thank goodness I kept my gloves on.* The elephant's trunk is about six to eight inches in length, about an inch and a half wide, *Ok!* As I take a closer inspection of the trunk, I notice something else. There are a few chips of paint missing from along the elephant's trunk. *Oh shit!* My patient may have retained some foreign bodies inside her vaginal area. I put the elephant down on the counter, blocking its view from my patient as I tried to get her attention. "Do you feel any possible material or substance that shouldn't be there in your vagina?" I ask as delicately as possible. In most cases, patient's feel foreign body sensation very well. If they don't feel it, it is usually not present. However, in my patient's situation, the extent of the swelling may hinder her ability to sense the FB present.

"Doc, I don't know. Why do you think something is in my pussy? The morphine makes me not care about the pain but I'm still afraid because it still feels like my pussy is multiplying. Now you're saying something is inside. Please get it out." She starts breathing fast again. The valium's effects are weaning.

"Give her another 10 mg of IV Valium. Pack her with ice and after we get some decrease in the swelling I need to make sure there aren't any paint flecks inside," I regretfully inform everyone.

I step outside the room and Dave, one of the night shift nurses, hands me a chart. "Doc, you need to see this guy right away," Dave stresses. Dave must be the earliest of the three night nurses that should be checking in for their shifts. He is a young, stocky guy that has a great even-keel manner. I can tell I need to hurry as Dave rarely gets this uppity. The chart reads: CC: Broke Dick 33-year-old male

10:03 PM

I walk quickly to Room 9. A deep voice is making guttural moaning sounds. The exam room door is open but I knock on the door as I walk in. "Hello, I'm the ER doc. Dr. Adams." I quickly notice Judy and another night nurse, Sharon. Sharon is the more seasoned of the night crew nurses. They are already getting an IV established. The two nurses along with the two in-house medics are circling the patient's bed. From the morbid patient's perspective, it is almost like circling vultures waiting for their prey to die. Or in reality, it is another patient misfortune from which we healthcare providers can get our kicks. I like extra help, but think my staff have become looky-loos. My patient is a large black man who is trying, but failing, to fight back tears. He appears to be naked except for a large beach towel covering his lower waist area. He is very muscular and probably taller than me, but with him sitting up in the bed it is hard to determine. When I refer to muscular, I mean ripped. This dude is chiseled like a bodybuilder. The idea of a guy who looks invincible crying has got me worried. *What is going on under this towel that can turn a superhero looking dude into a sniveling baby?*

"Doc, it's broken and it hurts something fierce." I figure if you are still reading this, you are not squeamish, so you will not react adversely when I tell you, yes, the penis can break. I reach down to the towel and realize today's shift has kind of a recurring theme.

"As soon as I see what we are dealing with, in seconds you'll have adequate pain medicine flowing in that IV," I try to reassure him. I am at the side of the bed holding the edge of the beach towel while looking in my patient's tear-filled eyes. All heads in the room turn toward my unfortunate patient's groin area. I gently pull back the towel as I see his eyes descend toward his own privates. "Don't look yet. It usually starts hurting worse when you see it. Wait until the nurse pushes some meds through your IV, ok?" He nods in understanding. Everybody else in the room was staring intently toward the big reveal. Nobody else was going to look away. They may regret that decision. Soon they'll have an image burned into their brains for all eternity. *I still do.* I pulled the towel down to his knees and instantly felt nauseous.

"Sharon, push 10 mg Valium and 2 mg Hydromorphone (the strong narcotic Dilaudid), hang a liter of NS, if he desats a little, just throw some Os on!" Basically, what I was saying was sedate him and if his respirations slow resulting in lower oxygen, I'm fine with that, we can give supplemental oxygen. My priority is making him comfortable. What I am looking at is medically worse than my Vagalien. Simply put, his penis now resembled a giant eggplant. This very well-endowed man probably snapped the midshaft of his penis when he was fully erect. The rare event of penis fracture only occurs with an erect penis. The two cylinders that fill with blood are called the corpora cavernosa and rupturing the outer lining of one of these two cylinders results in a fractured penis. With the extent of swelling, I have a bad feeling his urethra (the tube that urine flows out when leaving the bladder) might be torn as well. Urethra injuries are rare but can occur without having an erection. The dark blackish purple mass of swelling left the shaft of his penis wider than long. It was both devastating and anatomically mesmerizing. As I had alluded to earlier, his natural length would make an adult movie star envious. *Now with the amount of blood draining into his extensive shaft, it was a horror spectacle that was hard to comprehend what one was witnessing.* "Guys, get some pillows to prop his pelvis and some ice packs, keep him NPO (Latin nomenclature for nothing by mouth). He will need to go to surgery tonight." I look up to my patient and am pleased to see the medication has really kicked in. His eyes are droopy and his breathing has slowed considerably. Even with all his muscle mass, the medicine is taking its full effect. That leads me to believe he rarely takes medicine and thus has a low tolerance. Medicine will have a stronger effect on him.

"Doc, you say sometin about sugary?" He is slurring his words now.

"Yes, I will call the urologist. That is the dick doctor and he is going to fix you up. How did this happen?" I ask, knowing now I might get an unfiltered explanation. Strong IV medications will often sedate patients, but I have also seen it have a truth serum effect. In fact, I was once called as a witness in a criminal case debating if truth serum effects were admissible.

The case involved a young man who supposedly had broken into a few garages and stolen tools and other stuff. Somebody called the police and described his car. Soon the police were on his tail and a high-speed pursuit occurred. Thankfully, the thief ended up crashing his car without anybody but himself getting injured. The paramedics brought him in and informed me only about the car crash, leaving out the prior theft details. After a quick X-ray revealed rib fractures, I ordered a modest dose of IV morphine before he went to CT scan. The patient was in a good deal of pain. When the patient returned from the CT scan, a police officer arrived and asked me if he could talk with the car crash victim. I said he could, but I was suspicious about a possible splenic injury that might necessitate an urgent trip to the operating room. My radiologist called to confirm my suspicions about a serious splenic rupture. I was on the phone quickly with the surgeon and the OR was called into action. While I was out of the room, the patient gave the police officer a full confession and detailed all he had stolen. I ordered another dose of Morphine as the patient left the ED on his way to the OR. The patient made a full recovery, exchanging his spleen for jail time. Months later I was called to court. The defense attorney was hoping I would testify that the confession was not admissible as the patient was under the effects of Morphine. I advised that in my opinion, patients are more truthful after IV opiates. I couldn't speak about the legality of information given after being given IV opiates (the Morphine), but I did relay what the effects of those drugs may have on a patient. The jury sided with the prosecution and he was sentenced to jail. The defending attorney was hoping for a Hail Mary and I wasn't playing for either team. In general, I don't relish getting called to visit the court house. However, this being my first court case and having the jury members enthralled by my medical descriptions, I actually enjoyed that opportunity to get out of the hospital.

Let's return back to today's innocent, very unlucky patient. What information will he reveal following his administration of IV pain and sedation medication? I can see on his face he wants to give me his best rendition of tonight's earlier events. He is shaking his head, trying to clear away what I like to call "Foggy Head Syndrome." The medicine is fulfilling its main purpose by distracting his brain from his injury. "Oh, Doc it was so incredible until it wasn't! Oh, oh man! My new girlfriend, Doc. She was so horned up. Her little sis was going to prom yo. It made her so excited. She bought some massage oils and super-glide for us, hell yeah! Ah man Doc, we were doing it doggy style. Oh God, Doc! I'm pretty big, Doc, and I ain't never had a girl able to take my whole monster, you know. She was able and lovin it, we both were. We were both slamming. I love doggy. She would pull forward when I pulled back and then when I slammed forward she would slam back, in complete perfect unison, like we choreographed or sometin. We would get further and further apart before coming together harder and harder each time. Oh, I was about to explode when I fell out right before I slammed forward as she was slamming back into me. I wasn't in when we collided and I hit her ass bone or something. I heard a loud snap and pain like I ain't ever felt. Oh, man!"

Everybody in the room was on pins and needles listening to every word until he finished his story. The pain medication was working like a charm. I tried looking him in the eyes, but found I was having difficulty pulling them away from his broken member. *I hate to admit I was having a hard time turning my eyes away from a man's penis.* It was like my eyes were caught in a tractor beam. The horror of its sheer size accompanying the grotesque color and shapes was captivating.

With great effort I look away to meet his eyes and say, "Hey, when the pain meds start wearing off, let me or one of the nurses know and we'll hook you up with more meds." I gently cover up his eggplant monster, forcing my eyes from reestablishing direct contact. With the tractor beam disengaged, the rest of the room's occupants were able to resume their duties as well.

There was a knock on the door. "Doc, don't get comfortable. You have to go spelunking in Room 3 remember. Those paint chips aren't going to find themselves. Sally has everything prepped," Betty pipes in. She was continuing her role as being my ever chipper taskmaster.

"Thanks for the reminder. Tell them to get Dr. Wang on the phone. He is up in OR with our zipper patient. After I inform him of our second penis case, I'll go treasure hunting." *I guess. Wang should be done with that surgery.* I suddenly realize I sent up the rectal tear patient at the same time. The rectal injury was life threatening and would take priority, so Wang probably has not gone to the OR yet. On a weekend night we rarely would have enough staff to open two operating rooms at the same time. Sometimes after regular working hours or holiday weekends, emergent surgery cases stack up and need to be prioritized. Of course, life threatening bleeding trauma jumps to the top of the list. I'm not sure if a few hours makes a difference for my penile fracture patient, but I know if his problem isn't fixed, there is a high risk for erectile dysfunction to develop from these types of injuries. He should jump ahead of a patient with foreskin entrapped in the zipper. *Red leather zipper boy will not be making it to prom this year.*

I walk back into Room 3, trying to psych myself up to go where the gray elephant has recently gone before. *Argh! Chances are good some paint chips may still be inside, but even if I were dealing with a non-swollen vagina, this would be a challenge. The extreme swelling may make this impossible. How am I going to psych myself up and delude myself that I have any chance to be successful? Well, I'm not calling Big John for help until I at least give it my best attempt.* "Any improvement in the swelling?" I ask as I enter the room. The owner of the Vagalien is snoring. *Thank you Lord.* She has even fallen asleep with her feet in the stirrups.

Her husband lifts up the sheet covering his wife's waist. "Much improved Doc, but still looks rough."

That is what I was afraid of. *Well, here goes nothing but I hope to get lucky.* I sit down on a stool, trying to inspire myself up as I'm looking at the two labial flattened footballs before me. My nurse had foresight. Lying on the tray next to me is a pediatric speculum, a large amount of lubricant, and an assortment of long forceps. The Vagalien is so rotund it would not be able to eat a normal adult speculum. This exploration will not make it happy. *Where do I begin?* I look over at the husband, "How were you holding the elephant when you tried to arouse your wife?"

He picks up the elephant and demonstrates in the air, "Like this Doc."

"Ok, thanks! Hand it over if you would," I ask. Trying to get a starting point, I hold the elephant near my sleeping patient's vaginal area and realize I'm grasping at straws. Trying to line up where the chips may have flaked off is totally random. I'm only looking for excuses to delay my search.

I'm about to hand the elephant back to the husband when my patient wakes. "STAY AWAY FROM MY PUSSY WITH THAT!"

I nearly drop the ceramic elephant and stammer, "I'm sorry. I was looking for a frame of reference to where the possible paint chips might be located." I was pleading. *I hope she bought it.* I didn't want to admit, spelunking in a strange woman's vagina for foreign objects isn't on my bucket list.

"Oh, please get them out. I'm sorry I'm freaking out but well, you know. Hell, it's staring you straight in the face, Doc." *I couldn't argue with her there.* Handing the elephant to the husband, I free my hands. Next, I lube up the smallest speculum in the department and begin. *I would like something to preoccupy my brain as well as my patient's attention.*

I begin my exploration and ask the husband, "What led you to use the elephant in the first place?" I figure he may be reluctant to share. Man, was I wrong. The next moment I felt like a priest receiving a full confession from a death row inmate. He started spilling his guts and didn't hold back.

"Well Doc, I had too much to drink at supper. I am usually fine if I only have one glass, but I drank most of the bottle of wine. Of course, I ran out of my Viagra last week. Even though I have a refill, like a dummy, I didn't get to the pharmacy before date night. Oh, God! Then we were kissing and shedding clothes in the living room. Oh, she was really wet and I was so limp. The sex toys are in the bedroom and I didn't want to walk all the way there and back. When I turned my head to reconsider walking to the bedroom I saw the elephant. It was next to the couch we were on. It was only an arms-length away. I wanted to get her off so bad. I totally blanked about her latex allergy and I didn't even stop to think about what kind of paint was on the elephant."

While he was rambling, I was having success. I had already removed two paint flakes and had spotted the third. *I was in the zone, the pussy zone. I always have great success when I'm* …. removing foreign bodies. I clasp the large, curved forceps over the third chip and exit my patient's cave of wonders. "Got all three, you can sit back and relax now. Things should start feeling even better soon." The next thing I do is complete the elephant trunk puzzle. I place each paint chip on the trunk in the missing locations to make sure all foreign material are accounted for. *Success!* I then place the fully assembled elephant back in its brown paper bag and crinkle it closed. I grab the bag and head toward the trash can. I was ready to throw this thing away. I was pretty sure nobody in this room would have any objections. I step on the garbage canister's foot pad to open the lid and...

"STOP! I want to keep it," my patient yells while sitting up in bed. Nobody in the room could believe it. I was about to ask why, but her husband beat me to it.

"Honey, why are we keeping it?"

She responds with a venom laced tone, "HONEY, if you ever put something in my pussy that doesn't belong there, that elephant trunk is going up your ass!"

I walk over and hand her the brown paper bag. "Give me a few minutes, I'll type up your discharge and write some prescriptions and if swelling continues to lessen, we'll get you out of here within the hour." I walk out of the exam room trying to shake away the Vagalien image from my mind.

"Doc, you are not going to believe it. I have good news and I have bad news. Good news is this will be the last patient I see with you as my shift ended at 10. Bad news is..." Betty hands me a new chart (Room 7). I quickly look away from her annoying sardonic smile and read the chart: CC: swollen private area 20-year-old female

You gotta be kidding me. I didn't know whether to laugh or cry at this point. "Betty, lead the way to 7 and hold the snarky remarks, please." To her credit, Betty holds her tongue. I think it was the first time all year. She realized that her shift was basically through and it is bad form to pour salt in a colleague's wounds when you'll soon be heading out the door.

"She looked really uncomfortable when I brought her to the room and told her to gown up. She didn't tell me specifically what was swollen, but pointed down to her crotch," Betty remarks.

"Well, I don't think it can top what we have already seen tonight," I respond.

We knock on the door and enter the room. A young woman was sitting upright on the exam table trying, but failing, to lean back into the head of the bed that was propped at a 45-degree angle. She was either too anxious or too uncomfortable to lean back. She had short black hair with distinctive silver highlights throughout. The silver in her hair matched her multiple earrings on each ear lobe and the single nose ring on her button nose. "Hello, I'm the ED doctor, Dr. Adams. You already know Betty. Betty will assist me with your exam and treatment," I add.

I could tell the sight of me didn't alleviate any of her worries and I continue to hope Betty's presence will have a reassuring effect. Her only response is a very quiet "ok."

I wait a minute to see if she would start talking more, but the poor young woman remains silent. Sweat is beading on her forehead and she is clenching her teeth. She looks to be suffering something awful, but is also embarrassed to be here at the same time. Her legs are pulled up into a butterfly leg stretch position. "Would you like to tell me or just show me the problem?" She answers by slowly lifting up her gown, revealing a swollen area of vaginal tissue.

Betty knows right away what it was. I need a few seconds to figure out what I was looking at. I bet the female reader knows what I failed to immediately recognize. Likewise, the male reader is still waiting for me to inform them. Of course, I knew what I was looking at. I am hoping I am confused for my patient's sake. Because, my poor patient's clitoris is enormous. More accurately, her glans portion of the clitoris is red and swollen larger than the size of a golf ball. The technical definition is "Priapism of the Clitoris." One could also call it an "Isolated Vulvitis," which is inflammation of the vulva (itis refers to inflammation). Vulva is the female external genitalia, which are the labia majora, labia minora, and clitoris. Her labia was not affected, and in comparison it made the clitoris that much more enhanced. I had never seen an isolated vulvitis. My elephant trunk patient had a vulvitis vaginitis from the depths of hell, but her clitoris was only about double in size. I would never use the term "only" when referring to a double sized clitoris unless I was comparing it to this new extremely unfortunate woman. You remember how uncomfortable and psychosis-inducing the situation was for the ghastly elephant trunk patient? Simply put, the clitoris is the most sensitive area of the most sensitive area. This young girl was miserable, but tough as nails.

In order to fully appreciate this patient's clitoris predicament, I need to provide some education for the clitorally illiterate. Wise women refer to the clitoris being like an iceberg. Most of the clitoris is invisible below the surface, with only the tiny glans part that is able to be seen and felt. This section creates the head above the surface. The entire clitoris is actually three to five inches in length (7-12 cm). It is actually a wishbone shaped structure. When stimulated, the entire clitoris can swell, but only the glans portion is seen. It is usually about the size of a pea and contains up to 10,000 sensory nerve endings. This is twice the penis. The clitoris is so sensitive, some women are unable to tolerate direct stimulation and experience better arousal from stimulation of the surrounding area than direct clitoris contact. The variation of clitoris size has scant studies, unlike the penis size studies of which we get weekly updates. *Big surprise there.* I hope you are now more educated and understand the plight of my poor patient.

So, what causes Priapism? Well, before we get there, let's beat a dead horse, shall we. Let's start with the definition of priapism. If you do an internet search, *yeh Google I'm talking about you,* Priapism is persistent and painful erection of the penis. Ok, Google uses the *Oxford Dictionary*, let's forgive them. How about two medical meccas in the United States health-care system, Mayo and Cleveland clinics. Prolonged erection of penis is Mayo's quick succinct definition. A persistent and usually painful erection that lasts for more than four hours and occurs without sexual stimulation develops when blood in the penis becomes trapped, and unable is to drain. This is Cleveland Clinic's more thorough definition. The problem I have is they only refer to it occurring in a penis. I had never heard it was possible for a woman to have priapism. Women experiencing it is extremely rare, but it still happens. However, if a problem more often involves the penis, the clitoris takes a back seat. The stigma for women to even discuss the clitoris is astounding. What about when there is a dysfunction of the clitoris? The penis not only takes all the air out of the locker room, but every room. I was never taught that women could get this and felt terrible about my ignorance.

Now, noble reader you know more than I did after my first few years as a practicing physician. Well, at least about female vulvitis and priapism of the clitoris.

My silent patient still is withholding any details on how this problem transpired. I know major causes of a vulvitis are infection, allergy (my prior patient), cancers, and excessive friction. Priapism can occur most commonly with medication and rarely more severe trauma than excessive friction. Specifically, priapism of clitoris can occur with a simple scratch or increase of androgen (male hormone most common example is testosterone). Some examples that can increase androgen are the use of anabolic steroids, or developing polycystic ovary syndrome. The causes are crucial in order to provide the correct treatment.

Even though she is reluctant to share, I need her to give me the full story. "I can have Nurse Betty put in an IV and provide some strong pain medication. Is that something you'd like?" She nods at me. I continue with my questions, hoping she would start to open up. "Did someone drive you here?"

"My girlfriend did. She is in the waiting room. She is feeling really bad because she is the reason it's so swollen."

Great, she has started to open up. "Oh, can you tell me what she did and how long has it been swollen?" Betty is starting an IV and providing a slight distraction for the patient's current painful predicament.

"Well, we were, um, in bed this morning and she was rubbing me. She was more aggressive than usual, but I kinda like it rough. She rubbed so hard I got a bit numb so the second time she got out a toy and pressed and rubbed even harder. I usually orgasm when my clit gets really stimulated, but the second time I wasn't able. Tisha kept trying and trying, but then it started hurting. When the pain got really intense is when the swelling started. It's been swollen for almost 12 hours now," she concludes.

"Betty, give her 10 mg Morphine, 50 mg Benadryl, and 20 mg Decadron. Oh, also apply as much ice as she can handle." I start treating it like an allergic reaction, but it wasn't one. The swelling was triggered by excessive stimulation. I didn't know what would help more than ice and time. Benadryl, an antihistamine and Decadron, one of the corticosteroids, were a long shot. Like Solu-Medrol, Decadron is a strong anti-inflammatory medicine. I really wasn't sure what would help a woman that had excessive swelling isolated to her clitoris.

I had experience treating male priapism back during residency. The most memorable was a young black male with sickle cell disease. The saddest part being, he was my patient multiple times. I'm going to get a little text book here, but if you can stick it out, you'll gain some medical knowledge. Sickle cell is an inherited disease where red blood cells have a sickle shape. The human body changed the genetic code of hemoglobin to protect itself from malaria. The benefit arises when an individual has the sickle cell trait (SCT). That means having one normal gene and one sickle cell gene. SCT is an example of a balanced polymorphism. That is a genetic change that has benefits and detriments. However, when someone has two copies of the sickle cell gene they have Sickle Cell Disease. Sickle Cell Disease not only lacks malarial protection, but can cause a lot of other medical maladies. Sickle cell trait can be good (where malaria exists). Sickle Cell Disease, not good at all. End of lesson.

One of those not good things that arises (*yeah*) from sickle disease is priapism. The first time I saw Marvin, the urologist was holding a syringe that was aspirating blood from his penis. The 16-gauge needle was inside the corpus cavernosum pulling blood out. He was on a morphine drip, as his over eight hour erection was excruciating. He was seventeen at the time and whenever he had a sickle cell crisis, it manifested as priapism. Sickle cell crisis is when those with Sickle Cell Disease have an acute painful attack. These attacks are very painful and the emergency physician needs to provide relief. We order blood tests that can aid in determining if a crisis is occurring, but there is no definitive test that is 100% in saying a patient is experiencing a crisis. We have to trust our patients when they say their pain is unbearable. Pain crises can occur in the chest, back, or any extremities. In all but one location it is not visually obvious. Marvin was an exception. I've encountered patients who could rival De Niro or DiCaprio for an Oscar, but even those great actors can't fake a six-hour erection. When Marvin came in, there was no acting involved in his presentation. Unfortunately, his prolonged erections occurred on a monthly basis. The third time I took care of Marvin, he had turned eighteen and was totally exasperated. He had developed a phobia with every erection during a sickle crisis or not. The fear associated with every erection possibly prolonging and necessitating an ED visit made him desperate for any solution. He was seriously contemplating having his penile muscle removed and a penile implant placed. Last time I saw Marvin, he had decided to put off surgery but hadn't ruled it out.

Well, I brought up Marvin as he was my only frame of reference for this problem. We physicians recall our prior experiences almost every time we treat a new patient. *I hope some of the treatment I ordered has had some positive effect on my girl.* After an hour of ice and letting the medications take effect, Nurse Sharon, who had taken over care from Betty, gave me a status update on my young woman's swollen lady part. "Doc, swelling is less, but Morphine is wearing off. Her anxiety is up a bit, but I think it might have something to do with the fact that her girlfriend is now in the room with her," Sharon informs me.

"Great, repeat 10 mg Morphine and Ativan 1 or 2 mg IV depending on her response to the Morphine. I'm going to touch base with Big John and see if he has other recommendations and can lay eyes on her." When Big John eventually saw my young woman, her swelling had decreased by half. At half her prior size, it was still the largest clitoris Big John had ever seen. We decided to send her home with pain control, continued antihistamines, oral Prednisone, and ice. Big John instructed her to avoid any direct area contact until he reevaluated her in his office.

There are many lessons one can take home about the three most recent cases. Prior to opening this book, I hope you had already realized how incredible the human body is. Now, you have been witness to pushing that body past its comfort zone to the breaking zone and in one case through that zone. Accidents happen even when we are careful, but negligence while attempting to obtain or give an orgasm should be avoided. Nobody wants an orgasm that results in an ER bill. After all, a pricey orgasm isn't necessarily better than a free one. To this day I still have the Vagalien image burned in my memory banks. It is not an image that enhances my libido. When I look back now, the correct course of action to avoid that orgasm gone bad, is even more obvious. *That damn lazy husband should have used his tongue.*

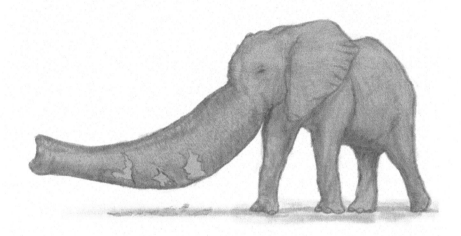

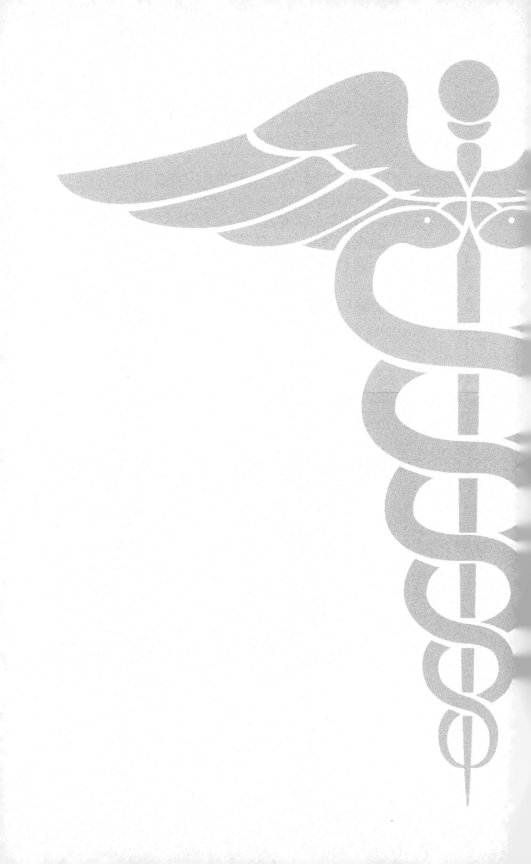

CHAPTER 5

Wrong! 10:40 p.m.

I pick up the Room 8 clipboard and read the verbatim description of the presenting problem. CC: ripped ball sack. 10 y.o.

Some triage personnel type a medically appropriate description of complaint. Others always write what comes out of the patient's mouth word for word. Even though "laceration to the scrotum" is medically more proper, in this case, there really isn't a pleasant way to describe this problem. I make my way to Exam Room 8 and hope the nurse has saved me and the patient some time by pre-medicating. Depending on each hospital's established triage standing orders, nurses can do a lot without doctor's orders. This includes simple giving Tylenol or Motrin for children presenting with fevers, swabbing for flu or Covid, ordering an X-ray, getting IV fluids started on a patient, and drawing labs. More specifically for my patient in Room 8, this would be applying a numbing gel to the lacerations to save time and decrease pain before the doctor even sees the injury. Some nurses are excellent at taking charge and not waiting for every little doctor order. However, some nurses don't want any extra responsibility and are afraid to be yelled at or disciplined if they do something wrong. In the later nurses' defense, there are idiot doctors who yell or call out a nurse for doing something they didn't want done, even when it was a totally correct thing to do. Some doctors always want to be completely in charge. My opinion of these particular physicians is simply they are assholes. I'm harsh because their actions have negative consequences for my work day. Nurses who are belittled or ridiculed are less eager to put themselves in that position again. In every work environment, it takes time to build rapport with your fellow workers. In a life and death workplace, it is essential to have your colleague's back. One can't just say they'll protect their workmates. They need to prove it. For instance, my nurse orders a hand X-ray on a patient waiting to be seen. However, after I evaluated said patient, I realized a wrist X-ray and not a hand was needed. I don't disparage her attempts or get upset. I add a wrist X-ray order and move on. Let me share an even stronger example of having my coworkers back. I once ordered IV Valium and IV Morphine on a back pain patient and my nurse mistakenly medicated the neighboring patient located next to the one for which I ordered the med. Doctors make this error way more often than nurses. This time the nurse had made the mistake. My nurse was distraught and came over to apologize and ask me if I wanted to call the supervisor to report his error. I picked up the chart of the patient who received the wrong medication and simply wrote the same IV Valium and IV Morphine orders, an exact copy of my previous orders. Both patients did fine, and my nurse knew I had his back. *Selfishly, I know it improves the chances that they have my back as well.*

Nurse Sharon is standing at the bedside of a young, scared boy. "Doc, I already applied the LET (Lidocaine, Epinephrine, and Tetracaine) gel, and I'll grab the suture kit. It's not deep but it is a little long," Sharon states. LET is a topical anesthetic, great for numbing areas that need stitches. Some non-medical people may be more familiar with EMLA cream, also a mixture of local anesthetics. Not that many years ago, my ED used TAC—Tetracaine, adrenalin and cocaine. Yes, the illegal addictive stimulant nose candy.

I see an older man standing on the other side of the bed, appearing too upset to sit in either of the two chairs along the wall. "Hi guys, I'm Dr. Adams, and I'm sure Sharon told you how the numbing gel works. Are you dad?" I ask, looking at the distraught man pacing on the other side of the patient bed. The man nodded. He was in a dirty white t-shirt and blue jeans. I looked at the boy. He is lying on the exam bed in a Scooby Doo t-shirt and a white sheet draping his lower half. "Well, who wants to tell me what happened?"

The dad stops pacing and starts talking. "Mikey was riding his bike in the dark when I told him not too. But the reason his sack is ripped up is because his bike seat fell off yesterday. He continues to ride around with just the seat post and no saddle."

I visibly wince, imagining the risk to one's private area with no bike seat. The boy is lucky he only has a laceration and not the beginning of gender changing surgery. "Mikey, is the numbing medicine helping? We can also give you some liquid medicine to swallow if you want."

Mikey responds, "Oh, it never hurt that bad, only I was scared. It is starting to feel kinda warm and less stingy now."

"Good to hear. I'll come back in ten more minutes and stitch it up. That will give the numbing medicine more time to work," I inform them. I head out to see the next patient.

Room 4 clipboard: CC: Abdominal pain 18-year-old girl

Often a patient with abdominal pain needs blood work and urine testing and often an imaging test, such as X-ray, ultrasound or CT. Belly pain patients often have longer work-ups than most other ED types of presentations. So, getting things started with a new patient before suturing my young boy's scrotal injury is a common way to keep efficient through any

ED shift. Also, I can limit the time of suffering by ordering pain medicine sooner on new patients.

Hurrying into Room 4, I see rosy-cheeked Melody with her beach ball pregnant belly starting an IV on a young woman. Melody's face continues to get more red as her shift prolongs because the baby in the oven keeps the heater on high. I look toward the patient again and I pause at the door trying to figure out what indeed I am looking at. The young woman looks like a princess. *This is surreal.* The combination of Melody's flushed red cheeks plus her opened white lab coat make her look like a cherub. No regular scrub top could hope to cover her large protruding tummy, so she wears a white lab coat that increases her temperature even more than her extra passenger does alone. *This patient is mesmerizing.* Lying in the hospital bed is a young blond beauty wearing a golden crown and dressed in a matching gold shoulder-less prom dress. This young woman is hypnotically stunning while adding to the fact that I have never taken care of royalty. *My rotund angelic nurse is taking care of a fairytale princess.*

"Doctor, my daughter has something seriously wrong with her," says the older and equally attractive woman in her own right, standing next to the patient. *The queen?* The patient's mother was wearing a shimmering long golden dress. My guess is that she was one of the parent chaperones at the prom.

"Oh, hello. Dr. Adams at your service, ladies. Can you describe what you are feeling?" I acknowledge the mother, then quickly stare at the patient, awaiting her response.

"Doctor, my lower left groin has been sore all day but continues to get worse. I thought I could tough it out until prom was over. After I got awarded prom queen, they put the crown on my head right before I threw up and passed out as the pain was so bad."

So, my princess was crowned the queen of the prom. This girl does not want to be in my ED unless she is dying. This usually means that there is something seriously wrong and probably needed to be accessed much earlier. I quickly palpate her belly and she jumps when I press in her lower left abdominal upper pelvic area. *Thank God,* she is holding a vomit bag and has perfect aim. She retches an enormous amount of dark green clumpy yuck, filling the entire vomitus bag to the brim. It occurred seconds after I pressed onto her left lower abdomen. The beautiful maiden has green goop dripping off her lower lip. To make things that much better, the goop's stench is similar to rotting roadkill.

"Melody, start some fluids. I'll order some pain and nausea meds. I'll come back to ask more questions after we can get her more comfortable. We will need to do a pelvic exam, but not until we get her nausea and pain under control," I instruct all three women.

As I'm heading out the door, prom queen's mom yells to me, "My baby is really tough and can handle pain. Something terrible has to be happening to her."

I don't want to discount the patient's mother, but she brings up a vital emergency medical issue. That issue being a person's PAIN. I think this is an appropriate place to discuss the most universal thing an emergency health care provider does. That is to take care of a patient's pain and suffering. Before we go further, I want to bestow a pearl of wisdom. The mother of our current young girl describes her child's pain tolerance as exceptionally high. This might be true and it is ok if someone speaks for you about your toughness in regards to ability to handle pain. However, I strongly advise you, never, I repeat NEVER TELL AN EMERGENCY HEALTH CARE PROVIDER THAT YOU HAVE A HIGH PAIN TOLERANCE! Why, you ask? Well simply put, emergency department nurses and doctors are acute pain specialists. We are not given that description, but that is indeed what we are. Of course, there are locations called pain clinics and pain doctors who deal with chronic pain. Unlike them, we see people on the worst day of their entire lives and people's most painful experiences ever! This can range from excruciating black widow spider or poisonous snake bite, difficult kidney stone passing, herniated disc in spine, crushed, broken or torn off fingers or limbs, heart attacks, brain and belly aneurysm ruptures, arrow or bullet body penetration injuries, and motor vehicle crashes that leave mangled bodies agonizingly clinging to life. That was just Wednesday's shift. The point is we don't deal with pain every day. We deal with pain every second of every day. The emergency department nurse who has over two months experience already has a good idea when any presenting patient problem is truly painful. Give them a few years and they know close to 100% certainty when a patient has a truly painful health issue. Well, Doctor, you are not being fair. Pain is subjective. This is true, but treating a sore toe or a tummy ache the same as a severed foot and a gangrenous bowel is never proper care. In fact, let me give you some numbers. I have had about 65,000 ED patient encounters during my career. I would say at least twice a week, if not daily, a patient tells me how tough they are and that what pain they are experiencing must be bad because they can handle most pain. Of those that said they were tough and able to deal with pain, only five or six patients in twenty-five years were what I would say, "TOUGH!" Those who are truly tough don't need to state it. Let me repeat that. Those who are truly tough don't need to state it! Actions speak louder than words. Or more specifically, in the ED, not having an overreaction to an excruciating medical problem speaks loudly. ED nurses and doctors want to limit pain and suffering. Remember we take care of pain not every day but every second of every day.

Let me share one of the few examples of a patient telling me that she had a high pain tolerance and proving it. A few years out of residency I rendered care to a nun in her mid-sixties. She had fallen down two stairs and broke her right forearm. She arrived in the ED wearing her nun habit outfit with the middle portion of her right forearm bent 90 degrees. Remarkably, the skin was intact and her pulses were still strong. I told her my nurse would start an IV so we could provide pain medication and after the X-ray we would give sedation meds so I would be able to reduce, which means straighten, her broken arm. She looked into my eyes and said, "Oh, Doctor, I'm pretty tough and won't take anything stronger than an aspirin. I don't need or want the IV. Thanks though." I remember looking at my nurse with her mouth ajar and shaking her head no. Like me, my nurse had no desire to treat the patient without giving pain medicine first. We both wanted her to have the IV medicine badly. Looking at the unnatural angle of her fractured arm was causing us pain. My nun once again reassured me before I did the reduction procedure, saying she can handle any pain. I relocated her arm perfectly, as God and this nun were my witnesses. In doing such, the fractured bone edges made grating noises loud enough that the neighboring patients could hear. My tough nun never moved an inch and her facial expression never altered. After a post reduction X-ray confirmed my excellent alignment, I splinted her arm. After finishing, I asked her how painful it was. Her response I'll never forget. It was a nonchalant, "Oh, I felt it. Now it feels better."

A few other memorable encounters of patients who stated that they are tough and proved it were a few military special forces patients. They didn't need to say they were tough, but at the time I was a young doctor and my guess is that they didn't realize I was more experienced than I looked. They had me reduce dislocated joints without taking any medicine. They are trained to deal with pain differently than normal humans. However, future patients that tell me they are super tough and can handle pain will be compared to prior patients who have said those same words and proven it. Pearl of wisdom when visiting ED: Unless you are as tough as my nun was or can rival a Navy Seal, keep your opinion of your toughness to yourself.

Slightly different but shall I say, in a similar vein, is the pain scale question. This is when patients are asked to rate their pain on a one to ten level. This isn't a measure of how tough or weak a person is, but what the current medical problem feels like to them. The majority of the time, a nurse is asking this question. Another pearl of wisdom is don't think the higher the number you tell the nurse will allow you to receive better or faster care. In fact, the opposite is more likely to occur. Patient's biggest mistake is to give a number past 10. Don't do this! You'll piss off the nurses. Most doctors, me included, medicate patients based on our nurses recommendations. Universal pearl #2: Don't piss off your nurse. Giving a number higher than 10 on a one to ten pain scale will piss off your nurse. Granted, people experiencing pain are often not thinking clearly. I'll repeat myself again, nurses and doctors want to limit pain and suffering. We don't like seeing patients in pain. We like providing relief and making people feel better, we really do. Remember, almost every single patient is asked to give a number for their pain when they arrive in the ED. A good rule of thumb is if you can say the number "10," you are below a 10 on the pain scale. In actuality a "10" is when you are incapacitated by pain. Those that are truly at a 10 are driven unconscious by pain, or nearly so. On the rare occasion (nurses usually perform this duty) I ask a patient to give me a pain number, I describe the number 10 differently. I tell my patient "0 = no pain and 10 is so bad you would prefer to be dead than continue to feel what you are feeling for another minute." On the rare occasion when someone gets under my skin and I respond like a jerk is usually after they give me a number above ten. I reiterate: "That means you would rather be dead?" If they say yes, I respond: "I can make that happen!" Then I assess their response to what I just said and if it actually registers, I downgrade their number. If it doesn't register, they are either crazy or in crazy pain, which is another topic of its own.

Before we put this topic to bed, let's address one final point with regards to describing one's pain. Patients not only get confused when experiencing pain, but also with understanding the definition of terms that describe their pain level and how well they deal with any pain. Those words are "tolerance" and "sensitivity." Surprisingly, many people fail to grasp their meanings correctly when those words are associated with pain medication. If someone says to the doctor or nurse, "I have a high tolerance to pain," chances are they meant to say, "I have a high tolerance to pain medication." The former means you can deal with pain, like my nun with a broken arm. My nun had a high tolerance to pain, and most likely a low tolerance to pain medicine. She most likely has what would be called a very high sensitivity to pain medication, low tolerance. She would have been snoring with a small dose of morphine. People who require high doses of pain medicine for mild injuries have a high tolerance to pain medication, a low sensitivity to pain, the opposite of being tough. As a patient wanting to inform the nurse or me as your doctor that you really want something for pain, it would behoove any patient to simply say, "I am a wimp and require high doses of pain medication to have any effect on my pain." All joking aside, I am being sincere when I say the patients who admit they don't handle pain well get more respect than the individual who says, "I'm really tough and have a high tolerance to pain." Bottom line—piss the nurses off and your bad day may continue. Endear yourself to the nurses and you will be rewarded.

I make my way back to Room 8 and the young boy with the scrotal injury. The numbing cream should have had ample time to ensure its full anesthetic effect. The majority of the time, and in this case, I will still inject more anesthetic. The topical effects will make injection less painful. Occasionally, the gel is all that is needed before suturing. The location and the size of laceration determine if I add lidocaine via a needle. If the area is more sensitive and the cut is long, I infiltrate additional local anesthetic. Sharon has a laceration tray all set up including a small bottle of lidocaine. "Hi Mikey, you doing ok buddy?"

Mikey nods. Dad is still pacing on the opposite side of the bed from me as I sit down on my stool and slowly roll toward the edge of the bed. I lift off the towel draping his private area and expose the cut by removing the numbing gel coated cotton ball. His scrotal laceration has a nice circular blanched appearance. The paler area of skin is an initial confirmation the numbing gel infiltrated the surrounding tissue. I still plan to infiltrate more as his injury is the entire length of his unfortunate torn scrotum.

"Dad I need you to sit down in a chair or step outside," I instruct what I thought left no room for arguing.

"I'm fine. I have no problem seeing blood. Just get on with it, Doc," is his flippant response back.

"I'm not kidding. If you don't sit down or leave, I want you to turn around and not look at your boy's injured area. I will not start unless you turn around and stay looking at the wall. I have other patients I'll go see and keep you two waiting," I retort, trying to keep control of my temper. Why am I so particular that he sits down or avoids looking at the wound? I have had family members on more than one occasion pass out when they see loved one's injuries being worked on. It has resulted in a new patient for me and a second ER bill for the family.

"Ok, ok, Doctor. I'll turn around and not look," the dad responds. I don't really trust his tone, but I've warned him and I hate punishing a kid for his dad's stubbornness. Nurse Sharon is gently holding one of Mikey's hands and resting her other forearm across his pelvis to limit any possible movement that may occur during the repair. I irrigate by flushing normal saline a number of times and Mikey slightly moves when he feels the cold water on the portion of his family jewels that wasn't numbed. After finishing irrigating, I drew up 3 ccs (3 milliliters) of lidocaine in a syringe. I then inject the small amount of lidocaine with a tiny 30-gauge needle into the cut just under the subcutaneous skin layer of his scrotal sack, Mikey doesn't budge. Nonetheless, I see a movement at my extreme peripheral field of vision and a second later Sharon yells, "SHIT!" as I hear Mikey's dad hit the floor with a loud THUD! The idiot had turned around to look at the exact time I put a needle into his son's scrotum and down he went. He took nearly ten minutes to wake up with a now large laceration across his head. I end up placing over a dozen staples in his scalp. During his laceration repair, each time he was about to open his mouth I uttered the phrase "Shut it!" After six or seven "shut it!" and threatening to staple his mouth shut, I finish stapling his head laceration. Mikey's wound was finished much earlier and with less fuss. It took me eight small sutures and Mikey was a perfect patient. I like to think Mikey's dad learned a lesson, but I know Mikey did. LISTEN WHEN THE DOCTOR TELLS YOU SOMETHING!

I shook off my anger over the previous unexpected case and head (*yeah*) over to see how the prom queen is faring. The unfortunate delay was not without some benefits. While stapling Mikey's dad up, prom queen's urine results and some blood tests had returned. She is not pregnant and does not have a bladder infection. She has an elevated white blood cell count that is not specific at all but is an abnormality. Some possibilities are crossed off my list but my differential is still extensive. She may be suffering from: an ovarian cyst, tubo-ovarian abscess, ovarian torsion, diverticulitis, bowel obstruction, pelvic inflammatory disease (PID) like chlamydia or gonorrhea, a flare of Crohn's, or Ulcerative colitis she hasn't had diagnosed yet, among other possibilities. I walk in and she seems to be doing much better. She is no longer wearing a crown, and replaced her prom dress with a hospital gown. The smile on her face doesn't appear exactly normal, but much improved compared to the vomit drool after spewing in a vomit bag when I last looked at her. Physicians and nurses are human and no matter how hard we try to suppress any attractions or arousals, even when we know they are completely inappropriate, they can happen. When I first put eyes on prom queen she made me catch my breath. An ironically beautiful thing with the ED is this. A quick change into a vomiting Exorcist-like person erases all traces of unprofessional thoughts.

"Things look to have improved some. Tell me more details about the pain. When did it start? How did it progress?" I look at the prom queen who gives me a strange smile and blows me a kiss. I then look to her mom to see if she noticed the air kiss. The mother was looking at me and started answering my questions.

"She has had some pelvic pain for months now, but the severe pain and vomiting started this morning. Her menstruation has never been consistent. Oh, you're probably going to ask next, so I'll just tell you. She has been sexually active for about one year, but she promises that she has used a condom 100% of the time. I found out this week and scheduled her first gynecological exam for next week. This will be her first pelvic exam. Right honey?" The mom looks down at her daughter and the prom queen blows her mom a kiss and then starts giggling. I was very confused by her reaction as I had ordered a dose of IV Compazine for her nausea and IV

Fentanyl for pain. People can respond euphorically to any narcotic, but something seemed off.

"Thanks. We need to do a pelvic exam and then I'm going to order a pelvic ultrasound test," I inform Mom and this lets Melody know that now is the time to position the patient in the stirrups.

Prom queen is in a vaginal exam position and something very awkward occurs right as I was about to insert the speculum. My young patient's tongue had started making suggestive movements at me. Then when I insert the speculum she starts moaning pleasurably. Her mom turns beet red and cries out, "Honey are you all right?"

I look at the patient's cervix and it appears normal. I look at Melody and nod rapidly for my culture swabs as I want to get this exam done ASAP. I finish in record time, pulling out the speculum, but needed to do the manual exam. Melody is ready with some lubricant and I quickly place my right hand in the patient's vaginal opening. My prom queen patient starts kicking her feet up out of the stirrups as I palpate the cervix. While I palpate the cervix, I look at the patient's facial reaction. If there is cervical motion tenderness, a look of pain comes across a patient's face. Prom queen has a distorted smile and actually says her first words since before she had vomited. In a dark deep voice that sounded much different than her earlier high-pitched princess voice, she says, "Keep giving it to me, Doctor." I try my best to ignore her by picturing her beautifully stunning face with green stinking vomit. I should have stopped then, but I really want to pinpoint the location of her discomfort. Trying to finish the exam as fast but not miss anything, I proceed to reach further with my right hand up into her left ovarian area and "OUCH!" the prom queen and I both yelled at the exact time. I touched the source of her pain and that source bit me. I pull my hand out faster than a kid moves his hand off a hot stove the first time they get burned. "Doctor, do it again. I want more! Mommy! Tell the doctor to move it." Prom queen wouldn't stop her sexual rambling with her deep possessed voice. Her split second of discomfort from my touching her pain center only revved her up more. If she wasn't talking, her tongue was protruding inches from her mouth licking the air rapidly. She started gyrating her pelvis and lifting her legs much higher than the stirrups. She was even waving both her hands toward her pelvis saying, "Come on in, move it. I like to move it, I need to move it. I like to move it!" She was singing the song from the Madagascar movie with the crazy lemurs. Her poor mom started sobbing. Melody's angelic face turned white with fright. I was flabbergasted.

With everything that was happening, nobody else realized I had actually been bitten by her ovary. I need to sum up all that had transpired. My prom queen patient had turned into a psychotically possessed hyper-sexual being with a masticating vagina, singing I like to "Move it, Move it." *What the hell was going on?*

When we encounter a patient with a plethora of medical diagnostic dilemmas, making sure we address and treat each one can feel overwhelming. We step back and create a problem list. Once we have that list we can start administering treatment, starting with the most serious issue and continuing down the list. This usually occurs with elderly patients taking over a dozen medications who present with not one or two acute issues, but five or more, in addition to their up to twenty or more chronic ailments, I am not exaggerating here. I now need to do this for an 18-year-old healthy woman. *Well or at least she used to be before the demon took control.*

My young prom queen's problem list:
1.) demonic possession
2.) ovary with teeth

3.) severe abdominal/pelvic pain

4.) vomiting

5.) high WBC count

6.) irregular menses

Let's address the most serious issue first—demonic possession. Ok, unless it is actually true demonic possession, then a likely surgical abdominal problem should be number one, but this particular list is ranked in order of most freakiest problem. Prom queen was not acting possessed when she arrived. This problem started in the ED. Even with there being a blood full moon, I don't think a dead wandering soul from a dark sexual demon was floating around the ED and decided to jump into our young woman. I might be mistaken, but I am pretty sure this is a problem I caused. The word that describes this is iatrogenic. It refers to an illness caused by medical treatment or examination. What medicines did I give her? Fentanyl and Compazine. Fentanyl, the strong synthetic opioid has made a lot of headlines recently, but it alone didn't cause her demon possession. Yes, narcotics can cause psychosis.

The nature of her psychosis leads me to believe our other drug selection was also involved. The IV Compazine most likely played a large, if not major role. It is notorious for many side effects. In fact, at this point in my career, I rarely use it. I probably order it by IV route once or twice a year. These few times are when a patient requests it because of prior good response. One of the most serious side effects caused by Compazine and contributing to our young woman's demon is akathisia. Akathisia was one of my favorite words I learned in medical school. I thought it sounded so cool. That is until I saw my first patient develop it moments after receiving IV medication to treat a problem such as vomiting. We replaced a problem with a much worse one. The patient stood out of bed, ripped out the IV, demanding to leave but not wanting to leave. He frantically paced around the room, spinning around like a demonic energizer bunny. They were talking a million miles an hour as if they had consumed 100 Starbuck coffees in the past minute, and legs jittered like they were squeezing every muscle from the waist down fearing he was about to empty a full bladder. His facial expression was one of pure overwhelmed distress, like your work deadlines for the next twenty years are all due in the next minute and your hands are free but your feet are tightly bound. This is what "internal restlessness" looks like and what akathisia means. The worst ones I've seen can be described as a panic attack going nuclear. Thank goodness I have never experienced it and I feel terrible when the medication I have ordered causes it. Most commonly it occurs with patients taking long term antipsychotic medication. In those they refer to it as a movement disorder with the inability to remain still. It is still akathisia, but develops over a longer time period than say, thirty seconds. Not to lessen the slower acting more chronic condition, but when it occurs seconds before my own eyes, I can feel my patient's pure nightmarish angst. My young prom queen's hyper-sexual speech component was unique to her. The Fentanyl probably contributed and may have helped alleviate some of the usual akathisia angst. However, the demonic-like movements where her hips and legs were thrusting and gyrating was similar to other patients I have seen who only received Compazine. The treatment is benzodiazepines, IV Valium (Diazepam) or IV Ativan (Lorazepam) and IV Benadryl (Diphenhydramine). I had Melody give her 10 mg Valium and 50 mg Benadryl in her IV.

Now for problem number two: the biting ovary. I knew what this was seconds after my hand was withdrawn to a point of safety outside the prom queen's vagina. As a resident, I encountered this before when I had done a pelvic exam on a woman experiencing vague lower abdominal pains. After doing the manual exam and telling my attending physician that, "I could have sworn I palpated teeth where her ovary should be," he surprised me by saying, "I believe you." We ordered an ultrasound and this confirmed what we suspected—a germ cell tumor of the ovary, a teratoma. What separates a teratoma from other tumors is that multiple tissue types are involved, such as hair, muscle, bone, and yes teeth. They usually are benign, but not always. However, their presence increases the risk of developing what is causing our patient's presenting complaint. What is causing our prom queen's severe pelvic pain, the third problem on our list? The answer is an ovarian torsion. The increased mass of the ovary caused by the teratoma led to the ovary being twisted on the supporting tissue. This twisting can result in cutting off blood supply to the ovary which causes severe pain and can lead to loss of the ovary. This is a surgical emergency. The solution for the ovarian torsion is getting Big John to take prom queen to the Operating Room. Once there, he'll remove the teratoma, solving problem number 2. Then he'll untwist the ovary, hopefully reestablishing proper blood flow, most likely solving all the rest of our young woman's problems.

I called Big John at the same time I ordered the ultrasound. I was very confident in my diagnosis even without the imaging. I also knew this tough silly young woman had waited all day suffering because of the chance to be crowned prom queen. Her delay in seeking medical treatment had jeopardized her ovary. The clock has been ticking and the lack of blood flow to the ovary may have been too long. I have to hope her lack of pain late in her care was from medication effects and not the demise of her ovary. Things hurt really bad when dying but when dead, pain actually lessens greatly. Simply put, after the tissue is dead, it no longer feels.

Big John actually wheeled her to ultrasound himself. Prior to pushing her bed, I introduced him to the prom queen's mom and gave him a quick recap of the hyper-sexual demon visit. Most importantly, I told him how long she had been suffering and he was as concerned as I was that the clock was ticking against her ovary. Dr. John told the OR crew to hold off on starting any of the semi-urgent cases. *Yup, poor red leather boy and his foreskin in the zipper is going to get pushed back again. I did use a lot of lidocaine when I numbed him up, but if he has to wait any longer, I sure hope Dr. Wang anesthetizes his poor penile tissue again.*

So, what happened to the prom queen's ovary? Her mother stopped through the ED later that night to tell us. She wanted to thank me and Melody for wonderful care and informed us of what transpired. She told me that Big John removed a 9 cm teratoma (4 inches) and successfully unwound the ovary in time. They decided to admit her for observation overnight because her breathing after taking her off anesthesia continued to remain shallow. When she did finally wake, she told her mom she was super embarrassed. Yes, she couldn't believe her improper hygiene, not her behavior. You see, the last thing she remembered was vomitus hanging off her lip and a terrible odor from her mouth. She hated herself for representing her school looking and smelling so horribly. Her mother was so relieved that her daughter had no recollection of her provocative hyper sexual antics. The beautiful prom queen might have no memory of her demonic akathisia actions, but because I will never forget, you were given a full account. You're welcome!

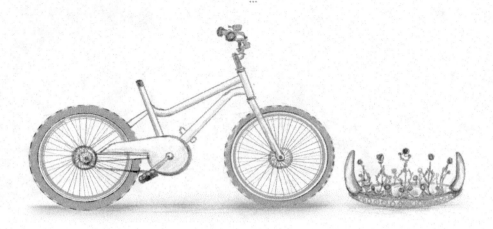

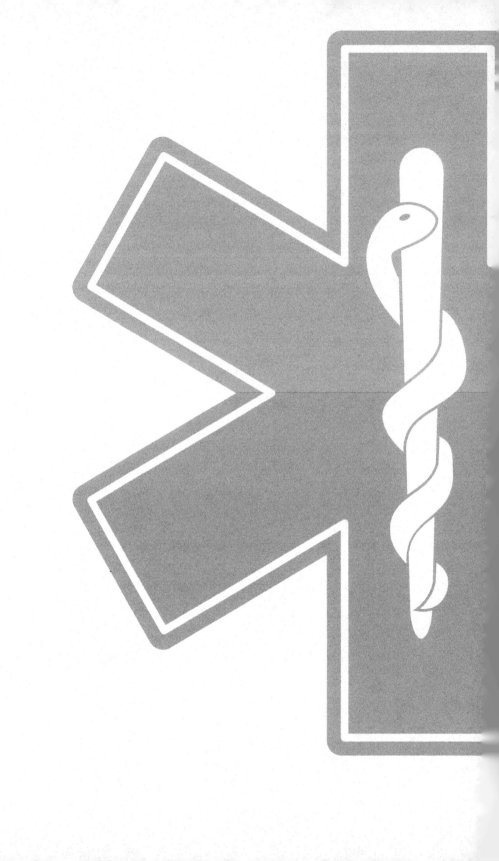

CHAPTER 6

Really Wrong! II:5I p.m.

Room 7 Clipboard CC: vaginal bleeding/pregnant 20 y.o.

As I walk over to Room 7, I start writing orders down on the chart. Bleeding while pregnant is a simple work up for the ER doctor. By definition, it is a threatened miscarriage. I order a simple urinalysis. A urinary tract infection (UTI) can cause bleeding, but even an asymptomatic UTI in pregnancy is something we treat. More importantly, I ordered a blood test that gives an amount of the hormone Human Chorionic Gonadotropin (hCG), called quantitative hCG. It is formed from placental tissue. The level in the blood can indicate how far along a patient is. I also have to find out the patient's Rh (Rhesus factor) blood type. It is only of concern if mom is Rh- (and baby happens to be Rh+). Only 15% of Americans are Rh negative. Old records may help or I can order a blood test. Finally, I often order an ultrasound. If she has already had one that confirmed an intrauterine pregnancy (IUP), I might not repeat one. However, if she never had one, it is important to make sure the pregnancy is implanted in the uterus. A pregnancy that plants outside the uterus, for example in a fallopian tube, is called an ectopic pregnancy. Ectopic pregnancies are life threatening. Another benefit of ultrasound is that a heartbeat can be visualized after six weeks versus 12 weeks to be heard with a doppler device touching the outer belly. Thus, ultrasound can provide information regarding if the fetus is still viable. The meaning of viable is the ability to live. Sometimes the initial ultrasound doesn't provide a definitive answer. The pregnancy is too early to see anything. Diagnostic and treatment aspects are easy. Dealing with the patient's emotional component, that's the difficult part.

I knock on the door and don't hear a response. Nurse Sharon arrives a second later. "Doc, she should have her gown on now. We should be safe to go in." I turn the knob and we both enter the room. A distraught young woman is lying on the exam table. In the chair alongside the table is an equally upset young man. "Hi guys, I'm Dr. Adams." These are emotional interactions and the best way I can lessen their uncertainties is by informing them exactly what will transpire. More surprises are the last thing they need.

"Are you in any pain?" I ask. She shakes her head, no. "How low have you been pregnant?" I continue my questions.

"Oh, about eight or nine weeks. This was my first. I lost it, didn't I?" she starts sobbing.

To his credit, her male partner embraces her and kisses her forehead. Then he mumbles to her, "It's ok, we can always try again."

I give them a minute and then I gently interrupt, "You are probably correct, but sometimes women experience lots of bleeding and don't miscarry. Have you had an ultrasound yet?"

She rubs her eyes on her boyfriend's shirt and then looks up to me. "No, I haven't seen my obstetrician yet. I have my first appointment next week."

"Well, let me tell you what's going to take place. We'll send off urine. Someone from the lab will do a quick blood draw and I'll order an ultrasound."

She looks up at me with her pleading eyes and asks, "Doctor, am I losing the baby because I did something wrong?" Her male partner also turns his face to stare toward me as he wants the answer to this question as well.

I don't know if it helps, but I have a go to line that I use during these all-too-common patient encounters. "If it is a miscarriage, it almost never has anything to do with what you have done, but often a chromosomal abnormality. A miscarried fetus has either too many or too few chromosomes, so it would not survive to birth anyway." I leave out the fact that certain lifestyle choices or other medical conditions also can result in a miscarriage. They already feel guilty regardless of the actual cause. Thus, this is not the time to throw them under the bus. "I'll come back and explain all the findings when they are resulted." As I open the door and follow Sharon out, I hear the young woman start crying again.

Both Sharon and I walk back toward the center of the ED. After we passed a few rooms, Sharon turns to me and in a matter-of-fact manner states, "That sucks, but I think her boyfriend is relieved. He already wants to try again and I think he is only putting on a show, pretending to comfort her."

I am shocked at her opinion. "You really think he wanted her to miscarry?" I respond.

"Doc, you are so naive. Neither of them had wedding rings. Pretty positive he doesn't want a baby. He only wants all the action he can get. A new baby will only limit his action. He's a pig, but not a stupid one."

Wow, did I miss something or is Sharon totally off base? Sharon is usually pretty accurate, but could I have been that oblivious? Well, that's the poor girl's issue not mine. I hand the order sheet for Room 7 to Cindy. The ultrasound tech should still be here as they barely finished verifying my ovarian torsion teratoma with Big John. So, I should have an answer soon. These are sad cases, but pretty dull as far as ED excitement goes. I see that I have another chart in the 'to be seen' rack.

Room 3 Clipboard CC: arm broken/fell off trampoline 6 y.o. male

I grab the chart and walk to Room 3. An entire circus menagerie is surrounding the young male patient who is abed. Three small active boys are scampering around the exam room. I am guessing they are boys because of their actions and mannerism, but all have long hair that makes their gender come into question. The frantic patient's mom is trying and failing to keep his three brothers still. The jovial brothers seem oblivious to their miserable looking older brother. The only one not moving is the teary-eyed young patient, sitting still trying to be tough with his left arm in an obvious kitchen fork deformity. His fracture resembles a fork with the prongs pointing down, the base of the fork jutting upwards. This can occur when a young person breaks both their ulna and radius of the forearm. When patients are young enough, the outer bone layer, periosteum, doesn't snap but stretches and kind of holds the broken bone fragments from separating completely. "Doc, I finished the IV and ordered the X-ray already. What do you want me to give him for pain?" Dave asks.

I look at my patient realizing if he weren't so big, I might have mistaken him for a girl because of his long hair as well. His bangs cover the upper half of his watery eyes and in the back his brown hair goes past his shoulders. At six years old, he looks nearly one hundred pounds. "Great Davey. Give him 5 mg Morphine. Hi, I take it you are mom to our unfortunate young man here?" I ask, looking at the woman who is trying to herd her other children.

"Yes, I'm sorry. My husband is serving overseas and it was too late to call a sitter. Tommy had to go out and jump on the trampoline after bedtime." The mother is a trim young woman with her hair tied in a long ponytail.

"I'm sorry, mom," Tommy starts crying a little more. I know his fracture hurts, but I think Tommy feels worse about putting his mom through all this hassle than the pain of his broken bones.

"I'm Doctor Adams, and we'll realign his fracture in no time. How long since Tommy ate?" I ask as sedation medicine can induce vomiting in patients that recently ingested.

"We had supper around 6PM. Tom, you didn't sneak any food later, did you?" the mother asks as Tommy shakes his head no. Jane the X-ray tech arrives with her portable machine and after Nurse Dave pushes some IV morphine, she takes the X-rays. It is one of those fractures that I really don't need an initial image other than for baseline and justification purposes. I need to justify the moderate sedation I am going to order.

"Well Mom, we have a great medicine that will allow me to straighten his arm and he won't feel or remember anything. It's called Ketamine." I usually give a spiel about Ketamine being a dissociative anesthetic. It detaches one from his body, but he is still awake and breathing. There are rare side effects and a scary elusive one termed emergence phenomenon or delirium. Because Ketamine is a hallucinogen, dreams and altered perceptions occur. Those are exactly why people abuse it to get high. The emergence problem arises post anesthesia either in the ED or when a patient gets home and suffers nightmares in their sleep. This is exceptionally rare and likely has no long-term effects at all. The mom continues to wrangle the three younger boys and seems very preoccupied.

"Whatever you think, Doctor. I trust you," she sputters, scooping up the smallest boy. She seems happy to have one contained and content to let the other two tire themselves out on their own. The mom sits down in one of the chairs with the smallest child now in her lap.

"Davey, get the consent for mom and I'll order the Ketamine and the post reduction X-ray. Tell the respiratory tech we have a sedation in five minutes. Get Javier to bring in the ortho cart." Javier is helpful when extra hands are needed, especially when splinting fractures. Javier has been around for decades, so they tell me. He helps with splinting, EKGs, cleaning patients, or getting them dressed or undressed. He is the go-to gopher for anything. His positive, helpful, and his can-do attitude is a blessing to have every day. Even on days when the proverbial shit hits the fan, Javier's demeanor is constant. The only thing that has changed since I've known him is his goatee. When I arrived, his goatee was brown. Now it is a dignified silver. He also speaks fluent Spanish, which can be beneficial when we need an interpreter.

Everybody is assembled and I am about to tell Dave to push the Ketamine into the IV. Whenever I use Ketamine, I instruct the patient to think happy thoughts or even picture a dream vacation before we give the medicine. "Tommy, do you have a favorite sport or pet you love to play with?" I ask.

"Yeah. I like playing catch with Toby my dog. We also play soccer together," Tommy says while forming a smile for the first time.

"Good. Think about playing soccer with Toby. Davey push the Ketamine," I order. In seconds, Tommy's eyes go spacey and start to involuntarily move back and forth horizontally. This is called nystagmus and is pretty common with Ketamine. Tommy's mouth is slightly ajar and I reach for his arm. Javier already has the splinting material measured and ready. I pick up Tommy's broken arm and he doesn't notice. I then pull forcefully on both ends of the fracture and align the bones back where they belong.

The trick with any painful procedure in the ED is not to hesitate. Be it a fracture or dislocation, removing foreign bodies, large lacerations, lumbar punctures, or chest tubes. I learned early on that the only time I had any issue hesitating was if the patient felt discomfort. Achieving good anesthesia or pain control allowed me to have no fear and get what I needed done without delay. Probably the best example of this occurs with placing a chest tube. A chest tube is placed to simply drain fluid or air from the chest. It is a painful procedure and often needs to be performed rapidly which can limit good local anesthesia or sedation. Many times, the patient's injuries also necessitate need for intubation. Like most ED physicians, I plan to do both procedures simultaneously, or as close together as possible. When I slice the chest wall and puncture through the pleural space to basically place a garden hose in a person's chest cavity, it can be daunting. However, if they are unconscious from injury or our strongest medication, my qualms are gone and I can charge full steam ahead. As with anything in life, if one does the correct preparation, they can commence with their charging in. The proper dose of Ketamine for Tommy allows me to leave any apprehension at the door and straighten his broken arm in no time.

Tommy's brothers stopped running around during the procedure. They stared at their brother's bent arm. They were mystified how he allowed me to not only grab the broken limb, but manipulate it. They winced at the slight crepitus of bones grating that occurred when I aligned the fracture. The mother even placed the littlest boy down in the chair and stood up to move Tommy's hair out of his eyes. Javier and I splinted the arm and adjusted a sling over his shoulder. "Doctor, is it ok if I cut Tommy's hair? He refuses to stay still for me, that is why his hair is so long. He is actually the most rambunctious of all of them." *Wow, he is worse than his brothers? This unfortunate woman. If the Ketamine can assist her with a haircut, why not.*

"Yes, start cutting now as the medication may wear off soon," I answer. Leaving the room, I was impressed that the mom thought about cutting her son's hair. *Two birds with one stone. That stone is wonderful Ketamine. With four wild boys, she needs to take any advantage with anything that comes her way.* Switching gears, I need to go check on the results of my miscarriage patient.

As I head to my desk to see if the lab and ultrasound have reported, the EMS radio goes off. BEEP BEEP BEEP. "Police on scene: 40-year-old woman took unknown drugs having varying levels of consciousness, possible cardiac arrest. 10th and Grand old town house complex"

I look out toward the opening ambulance bay doors and see Jason sprinting a few feet behind Kyle. I think to myself that I'll be seeing them shortly. Best try and discharge my two current patients before they arrive. If this is a young cardiac arrest, I'm going to be tied up for a while.

Accessing my test results, I see my vaginal bleeding patient in room 7 is Rh+, and her urine is normal except for some blood in the sample. Her quantitative hCG level is over 50,000 in the 8-9 week range like she alluded to. Unfortunately, like she and I figured, her ultrasound shows only slight tissue left in the uterus. There is no ectopic, but basically the findings show a nearly complete miscarriage has occurred. I can type up her discharge and then I need to let her know what everything shows, or in her unfortunate case, doesn't show.

I find Sharon on my way to give the unhappy news. Often having a nurse along not only provides support for the patient, but me as well. Selfishly, it allows me to leave quickly after giving the required information and letting my nurse handle any post emotional issues that may arise. That's further reason to support your nurses. They reciprocate especially when the doctor forces them in a position to do so. "Sharon here are the discharge instructions. Let's get this over with," I state, handing her the paperwork. Sharon steps behind as I lead the way. Heading around the corner to Room 7, I start thinking about what Sharon had said about the patient's not so sad male partner. *Well, if he isn't upset, then it should be easy for him to comfort her.* I'm trying to put a positive spin on his supposed apathy. With her having a rock for support, he can get her thinking toward moving forward and not dwelling on the past. We arrive at the patient's door and using my left hand, I knock. I really want to get this over with as fast as possible. I turn the doorknob with my right hand at the exact time I knock. I did not wait for a response. After all, this is an emergency department. Nobody needs privacy here. Pushing the door open, I am greeted with an image I had never seen in my ED before. My patient was getting some support from her partner, but not the support I expected. His hands were supporting the back of her head as he was thrusting his erect penis into her mouth. Neither one had heard me knock. A second later, Sharon walked in behind me and was equally appalled, but was quicker with a verbal response. "What the hell are you two doing?" Sharon bit into them. The supportive partner tried to stuff his enlarged penis back into his pants while his girl wiped her mouth. *Well, this wasn't the rock-hard support I thought he would provide her. To each their own.*

I decided to move along as if nothing strange had occurred. "The results show a miscarriage. Keep your OB (Obstetrician) appointment this week as scheduled and Sharon has some paperwork for you," I spit out. I quickly turn and walk out of the room. *They have already moved on, even faster than I did, which I didn't think was possible.*

After the couple left the ED, I walked over to Sharon. She didn't want to talk about the couple's extracurriculars at all. So, all I said to her was, "Your impression of that dude was right on target." With Sharon's disinterest in further fellatio talk, I went to find one of my male staff members. The idea of chatting with a female staff about what I recently witnessed didn't have the same ring to it. My male paramedics Kyle and Jason were out on a run. That left Dave and Javier. I needed a man's opinion on what had transpired. Suddenly, loud screaming permeated the entire department. It was terror laced and high pitched. The screaming had snapped me out of my recent visual imagery. *No time for fantasizing in the ED.*

Later that week I had the opportunity to discuss the inappropriateness of giving/accepting oral sex in a public location. I was hosting my monthly poker party. The group was made up of mostly healthcare workers. Dave and Kyle were there along with a pharmacy buddy, another doc, and two local police officers. A few other nurses and medics usually show, but they were working a shift that night. I brought up the image of my fellatio-giving patient on the previous shift. I didn't tell them why she was in the ED. At the time, it occurred I was so shocked that it didn't really have time to register. However, driving home after that night shift, the situation really started to bother me. I couldn't put my finger on what was truly bothering me. Was it the fact that the dude who should have been consoling his lady was so selfish to put his needs ahead of comforting her? Or was it the inappropriate location that had me perturbed? So, I asked my poker buddies where they would draw the line on accepting oral sex? I was also curious at what my police friends would condone versus partake in. After they all gave an answer, I then asked if they would be willing to return the favor to their partner in the same location. The answers weren't surprising. Most men are definitely more selfish than women. The one unique justification we agreed on dealt with the anatomical differences of the sexes. Me and my more selfish brethren were grasping at straws to lessen our cunnilingus exploration. Human male anatomy allows further extension than a woman's similar sex organs. In addition, the human female is almost always more flexible and can position herself for performing fellatio better than the reverse. However feeble the idea of using anatomical reasons to justify men's selfishness, remember those reasons can only be applied to precarious public places.

The screaming was coming from the other side of the ED in my young forearm fracture patient's room. I motored over to Room 3. My six-year-old with the now splinted left arm in a sling was in a state of terror. He continued screaming, "AAAAH!, HELP! AAAAH! NO NO GET AWAY! AAAAH!" It was horrible to witness. His mom was crying, with her hands on his cheeks trying desperately to console him. "AAAAH! AAAAH" he kept yelling as he was trembling and continued screaming. It looked as if he had stepped out of the shower as sweat was dripping off him. His three brothers were huddled in the far corner of the room shaking. Dave was at bedside and looked completely baffled.

"What happened?" I ask as I enter the room. I was looking at Dave and the mother to see if they had any clue. The one silver lining was his hair was short and no longer hid his eyes. Unfortunately, Tommy's eyes still had a spacey look but over riding it was a look of pure fear. His eyes no longer had any nystagmus, the pupils were now large and motionless. What was unbelievable with his screaming volume, was the fact that he actually wasn't fully awake yet. "Dave, give him 5 mg of Valium IV." Poor Tommy was experiencing an emergence delirium reaction. The possibly irrational fear of this type of reaction is what has limited emergency physicians in the United States from using Ketamine on adult patients. It is believed that adults have a much higher propensity to have this type of reaction. "Dave did anything happen when his mom started cutting his hair?" When I walked out after fixing his fracture, everything seemed calm and serene.

"Well Doc, the little boys were playing hide and seek under the bed and used the sheets to act like ghosts," Dave admits.

Oh no! "Mom, did they jump at him or try to scare him while you were cutting his hair?" I ask.

"Well, they were trying to scare each other and I was focused on his hair. I finished quickly and ran to the bathroom. When I got back they were in the bed sheets pretending to be ghosts," his mom divulges.

I looked over at the three young boys and one stood up crying. "Mommy, I'm sorry. I kept saying boogie woogie woogie at Tommy. I was trying to scare him because he was just staring straight ahead. I wanted to get him to move and so I kept trying to mess with him," the brother confesses.

I now know why Tommy had the reaction. Nurse Dave didn't fully comprehend the harm of scaring Tommy prior to coming off the hallucinogen. He didn't stop the brother from what was actually occurring. From Tommy's point of view, complete terrorization. I have to assume some blame. I should have warned Dave, especially with the number of young crazy kids in the room. Moving forward, Dave will not soon forget what he witnessed. *I sure hope Tommy doesn't remember.* The valium did knock him out and he rested quietly for another hour. Thankfully, when he walked out of the ED later than night, he looked fine.

"BEEP! BEEP! BEEP!" the EMS radio blared. "Medic One coming in with a 40 year old female, probable cocaine overdose. Combative with cardiac arrhythmia, heart rate 190, BP 200/120, hyperventilating, but good oxygen sats. Five minute eta, Medic 1 out!"

Judy picked up the EMS radio, pressed the intercom button, "ER copies loud and clear medic 1, see you in five, update if any changes, ER out."

I look at my nurses—Sharon, Dave, Melody, and Judy, "Ok guys, let's prep Room 1!" My paramedic Jason gave a great report. Working in the ED while they await their next ambulance call enhances their overall skills. Most importantly, they are aware of not only what we need to know before the patient arrives, but they know what transpires following that arrival. Most paramedics don't have the experience of seeing and treating patients throughout their entire course of care. This actually gives in-house paramedics something the nurses don't possess. They have seen the dwelling or scene where patients came from. Some doctors and nurses can obtain a good history from the paramedic who transports a patient. However, even if the nurse or doctor is very good, the transporting paramedic might know some home or scene information that is beneficial.

Rarely during a busy shift, a critical patient arrives when you have a clean house. By that I refer to the ED being empty of patients or patients who are on cruise control and not needing nurse or doctor focus. It is a luxury that allows the ED staff to put all their combined energy on the one critical patient in the department for as long as needed. All hands-on-deck approach happens when we call codes. We call code blue when someone has had a cardiac arrest and CPR is being performed. We have trauma codes, stroke codes, and respiratory codes. Those happen at any time during a shift. When they occur, everybody who is able arrives to help en-mass. Nurses, ED tech, lab tech, X-ray tech, and respiratory staff arrive until we determine what critical patient's needs are. Then slowly or quickly, workers head back to where they originated. On the rare times when the staff and I are not busy and get that serious patient, it actually allows us emergency medical providers to do what we do best without distractions. Usually, I have multiple patient workups pending, so I can't really focus 100% on the new emergency. During that rare clean house, when a serious patient arrives and you have no mental distractions and can have a singular focus, to put it plainly, it's awesome.

I hear the ambulance pull up, and seconds later the bay doors open. In front of the ambulance is a squad car and the two officers who brought eyelash boy in earlier step out. "Doc, didn't think we'd be back so soon. You haven't glued anybody else's eyes shut have you?" one of the officers says as they both laugh.

"Very funny. What have we got now?" I ask them.

"Well, Doc this one is a hot mess. We crashed a drug house that some of the detectives had been watching. Two of her baby daddies are the local drug kingpins and the detectives want to nab them badly. They caught their girl. They are a bit worried she'll not live long enough to give 'em up. She tried to hide all the cocaine when we busted into the house," the officer informs me. My paramedic Jason finally opens the ambulance doors. In the back of the rig, a frazzled Kyle is securing the monitor at the patient's feet. The patient's entire body is twitching. Her legs are outpacing her arms by twitching twice the pace as her upper half. The patient is a middle-aged blond disheveled woman who looks 50 even though they reported her as 40. She is fidgeting and not wanting to stay on the gurney. She is wearing a much too small thin t-shirt with obviously no bra and tight blue jeans.

"Guys, roll her to Room 1! Have you given her any meds?" I ask. Knowing if she looks like this after some medication, she is really in rough shape.

Kyle answers, "Doc, I pushed 10 mg of Valium but she pulled the IV at the same time. I got a second IV in as we pulled up. She is actually a little better, so I think some of the Valium got in."

Well, it is as I feared. She looks this messed up after already receiving some medication. "Sharon, grab 4 mg of Ativan and 20 mg of Valium. We are not going to be shy tonight," I inform everybody within ear shot. A mistake a lot of young doctors make is under-dosing. With giving too much benzodiazepines or narcotics, the biggest worries are that the patient stops breathing or blood pressure may drop precipitously. If you are not dealing with a trauma patient, fluids can easily correct the blood pressure issue. Breathing is also overrated. Yes, let me repeat that, breathing is overrated, as far as an emergency physician is concerned. In the ED, we can breathe for you. We have oxygen bags and ventilators. Once we establish a solid airway, we can breathe for patient's indefinitely. The key comes with establishing an airway. Once an ED physician feels confident they can establish an airway in any patient that walks, rolls, or falls through the door, *game on. Overdose away baby.* Medicating strongly is the more professional description. Sorry if I'm sounding a bit too cavalier. In situations when patients hurt themselves or staff by flailing, the time to put them down was long before injury occurred. Having confidence in establishing an airway enables the ED physician to not hesitate about taking complete control. Many times, I have had belligerent drunks or other highly medicated patient's refuse testing. If they present to my ED and appear to have sustained a serious injury, like a brain bleed or broken bone, *I become their daddy.* What I mean by that is, I assume responsibility and I'm going to do what is in their best interest. Patients who give me their name, date (within a day or two is acceptable) and location correctly, and if they can repeat back to me when I inform them of what injuries we might miss without testing, even if intoxicated, I deem clinically sober and free to make their own decisions. If they are not able to do that, I become their short-term caretaker. If the nurses or I start getting verbally or physically bombarded by a patient that's refusing proper treatment, time to shut them up. A tube through the vocal cords makes it impossible to talk, and allows us to focus on the job at hand. *Saving their ass!*

The patient quickly gets hooked up to the monitor and I nod to Sharon to push all the Ativan and Valium. Both drugs are benzodiazepines. The main difference is Ativan works quicker than Valium and its effects are shorter in duration. I want some improvement as soon as possible and for a prolonged period. Her twitching continues. *The damn twitching is making me uncomfortable.* The monitor is showing a peculiar rhythm. The rate is almost 200 and she has a possible arrhythmia versus an exorbitant amount of ectopy. That means extra heart beats that come from areas other than normal cardiac contraction center. I need an EKG to determine her actual cardiac rhythm. The nurses take off the patient's shirt to allow Javier to start attaching the EKG electrodes. My patient has a mosaic of tattoos covering the majority of her upper torso, sparing her breasts. She refuses to let the nurses remove her jeans. She seems very determined that her pants stay on, even with Nurse Judy offering a blanket to cover her lower half. This tells me she has maintained some cognitive ability. I need to find out how much. I look at her eyes, seeing her giant dilated pupils. The conjunctiva or whites of her eye are a bloodshot mixture of red with sporadic white traces. Unlike opiate overdose that gives pinpoint constricted pupils, cocaine dilates the pupil. "I'm Doctor Adams, Miss..." I wait to see if she'll give me her name.

Finally, after what seemed a long time she mutters, "Tina, my name's Tina. My chest is killing me."

Ok, now we are getting somewhere. The Ativan has probably had some effect. Javier prints, then hands me the EKG. Her rate has slowed to 170; it is a sinus rhythm with multiple PVCs, and premature atrial contractions (PACs). The extra beats are occurring in both ventricle and atrial areas. Her main QRS complex (the main portion of EKG that represents the depolarization of cardiac ventricles) is a lot wider than I would expect for someone her age. That has me worried that she could switch into a more ominous rhythm like ventricular tachycardia (V-tach) or the deadly ventricular fibrillation (V-fib). I look her straight in the eyes and ask, "What drug or drugs did you take?"

Her head looks all around the room and stops on the doorway. The two police officers are standing right outside the exam room, but in view of the patient. "I don't want to say," she reluctantly answers.

"Was it cocaine? You don't have to say, but can nod yes or no. That way I can help you and you never said you took anything," I urge her. She nods. Then, I ask if she took anything else and she shakes her head no. Ingesting only one drug is unusual, but I think in this case she took a lot of that one drug. Unfortunately, there is no antidote for cocaine overdose and her heart is pushing toward bursting. She may be lying in bed, but her heart is running a marathon at a 40-yard dash pace, all out. In addition, my guess is she already finished two marathons before she got here. It is only a matter of time until her heart gives out. "Let's give her 10 mg of Versed, then start a Versed drip." Adding the third benzodiazepine I have in IV medication form, I decide to go big or go home. *My shift is only half over so I can't go home.*

At the doorway, two serious looking gentlemen start conversing with my police officers. Both men are dressed in a semi-professional manner, wearing khaki brown pants and puffy sweaters. I look a little closer and realize the sweaters are not puffy, but cover the bullet proof vests underneath. Also, they both have guns holstered at their hips. These are two detectives in street clothes. This was the first time in my career that non-uniformed law enforcement visited one of my patients. *I feel scared and excited.* "Doc, when you have a second, we really need to talk with you," the taller of the two detectives states.

"Sure, one minute," I respond. The cardiac monitor continues showing the ectopy but heart rate and blood pressure are dropping nicely. My patient's twitching and jitters are slowing down considerably now that Versed is running in her veins. I walk toward the room's exit and motion to the detectives to move out of the patient's line of vision. *Her medical condition is not going to improve by talking with, let alone seeing, law enforcement.* We are now standing ten feet from the room entrance out of my patient's sight. We are definitely out of hearing range, considering she has Versed flowing freely.

"I'm Dr. Adams. What's up?" The two detectives are very imposing. The short one is my height and without the bulletproof vest, his chest is probably twice as thick as mine. His partner is not as tall as Big John, but could have given Arnold Schwarzenegger a challenge for Mr. Olympia back in the day. As if they needed more intimidation, these dudes were both carrying heat and gave the impression they knew how to use it.

"Doc, we think she may be stuffing. You need to do a cavity search," the taller detective continues to take the lead. When drugs are carried inside the body, we use two terms to describe this—stuffing and packing. Stuffing is scarier than packing. When drug dealers use mules or carriers to transport drugs, they plan and prepare. This preparation allows the wrapping of drug/product to be placed in a safe or secure manner. This is packing. Packing can allow contents to even sit in stomach acid for extended periods before containers break down. However, if someone does a rush job or wants to hide drugs quickly, they put them in loose wrapper or no container at all and this is termed stuffing. Stuffing often results in the drugs being absorbed into the bloodstream, often with serious consequences.

Depending on the drug, a massive amount absorbed all at once often leads to a fatal overdose. My other dilemma is I am not sure legally if I can do a cavity search without a patient's consent. *These officers aren't the type you want to refuse.* Bottom line, if my patient is continuing to absorb cocaine nonstop, she is likely to die. I need to do everything in my power to avoid that possibility. *Except, I don't plan to violate a patient without her consent. I need to persuade her to give me permission.*

"Ok, officers, give me a few minutes. You can listen, but make sure you stay out of sight." They really don't appreciate how sick she actually is. I quickly walk back to the patient's bed. Her eyes are glassy, but miraculously she is still awake. Often the best approach is straight to the point. "Tina, are you hiding drugs inside your body?" She looks at me and rubs her fingers across her lips. She is indicating that her lips are sealed. Strike one, but that is as good as a "yes" answer. However, I still don't know if she swallowed or put them in her vagina or rectum. "Tina, can I do a vaginal and rectal exam? Nurses Judy and Sharon will be here the entire time?" She shakes her head no. Strike two. Before I decide to swing for the fences, I step out of the room and tell X-ray to do a portable chest, abdomen, and pelvis. Her lungs sounded fine, however her heart was anything but. In addition, foreign bodies may show up even if they are not opaque. Often, large translucent objects can project shadows or become more opaque if the size is enough to affect the radiograph. I step out while the X-rays are being taken and ask the detectives if they have a female officer who can come and do the cavity search. They inform me that their lone female officer working tonight hasn't punched in yet. I don't know what the laws state now, but back then the police could do a cavity search without consent but needed a same sex examiner. They were pushing me because they didn't want to wait an hour. I quickly looked at the X-rays and saw her chest X-ray revealed cardiomegaly, a very large heart. This was most likely chronic and some of the readings on the monitor might not all be acute. *This is good and bad.* Good in that some of her problems didn't start today, but bad in that she most likely had a damaged heart before today's cocaine fueled escapade.

Looking at the rest of the X-rays, I see one subtle abnormality. She had a hazy mass-like object, not in her stomach, but in her pelvis. I now have near confirmation that my patient stuffed cocaine in her vagina. You know how they say don't screw with drugs or they'll screw you up. *She literally screwed the cocaine and the cocaine was now screwing her over!* The faint area on the X-ray looked rather large. With stuffing, the material has higher risk of absorption. *I can't wait an hour for the female cop.* This is a big bag and most likely a deadly amount of cocaine. I am pretty positive if this bag opens, she is dead, regardless of what treatment I can provide. If she would have swallowed it, my guess is she would have bypassed the ER and gone straight to the morgue. "Tina, I saw on X-ray that you have something in your vagina. Please can I take it out?" She shakes her head no. "It could kill you. Please, I want to help you." She continues to shake her head no. "Sharon, open the Versed and give a 10 mg bolus." I was going to knock her out and she wouldn't remember anything.

Unbelievably, Tina hears me tell Sharon to increase the Versed. Before anyone realizes, Tina pulled both her IVs out before we can increase the dosage. "WHAT THE FUCK!" I yell. I rarely use the F word at work. It's vulgar and unprofessional, but there are moments when you can't help it. This was one of those moments. "Tina you could die," I plead.

"Doc, can I talk to you?" Kyle, my medic, peeks his head into the room. I needed to decompress, so I walk out to see what the hell Kyle wants at a time like this.

"What's up, Kyle?" I didn't hide my annoyance.

"Doc, I heard you say "fuck." I've never heard you swear like that. Well, it is probably nothing but I think I might have something that can help convince her to let you remove the stuffed cocaine," Kyle says.

"Go on man! Don't leave me hanging," I implore.

"Oh, sorry. Might be nothing, but when the cops were bashing down her bathroom door, Jason and I were in her bedroom and I was checking out all her pictures. I'm pretty sure she has two boys. It looked like she lives with the two drug dudes and possibly had a kid with both of them. One pic was kinda weird, but showed her sitting with what looked like two boys, one on each leg and possibly the two baby daddies behind their respective kids. The men looked like their kids. What mom would want to die when she has two young kids at home?" Kyle concludes.

Kyle is absolutely right. "Thanks man! That is great info." I rush back into the room. I get into my patient's face and ask, "Tina, what are the names of your two boys?" That gets her attention. She starts crying. "Those boys will be heartbroken if they never see their mom again." She looks up at me and in a stone-cold sober voice says, "The nurse can restart the IV. I'm sorry." Next, she reaches down, unzipped her jeans, and pulls them part way down. Unsurprisingly, she wasn't wearing underwear. What is surprising is the fact that she reaches up inside herself and pulls not one but two baggies of cocaine out. I can't believe the amount. She had two mostly filled sandwich bags containing a white powdery substance. They are both sealed and seemed intact.

Judy restarts the IV and the Versed drip. A remorseful Tina was admitted to the ICU. She admitted to snorting and licking what she wasn't able to stuff in the baggies. Her chest pain improved as her heart rate slowed. She eventually had an echocardiogram, which is an ultrasound specific to the heart. The findings showed both chronic and acute dysfunction. She had prior damage to her heart from chronic cocaine use. That, coupled with the amount she ingested, flared up her underlying cardiomyopathy. Tina eventually went to jail. I like to think she cleaned up and became a good parent. Truthfully, sometimes it is safer not knowing the outcome. What I did now was satisfying enough. My patient lived and as a bonus, she removed her own foreign bodies.

This chapter reflects many patients who present to the ER. Poor decision making resulted in an ED visit. Often, we encounter people who make the same pitiful choices over and over again like my patient, the cocaine stuffer. Those choices frequently lead to worsening short- and long-term health problems. Or in her case, jail and nearly the morgue. Other times, a playful decision seems innocent enough, but minutes later turns into a scary life lesson. The example of the fun act of scaring your older brother turns the family trip to the ER into a nightmare. Lastly, trying to turn a frown upside down by giving or receiving sexual gratification isn't a bad decision, but if you pick the ER for that location, then it is REALLY WRONG!

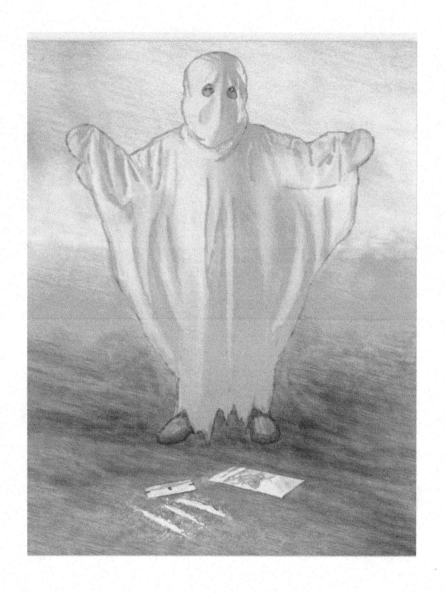

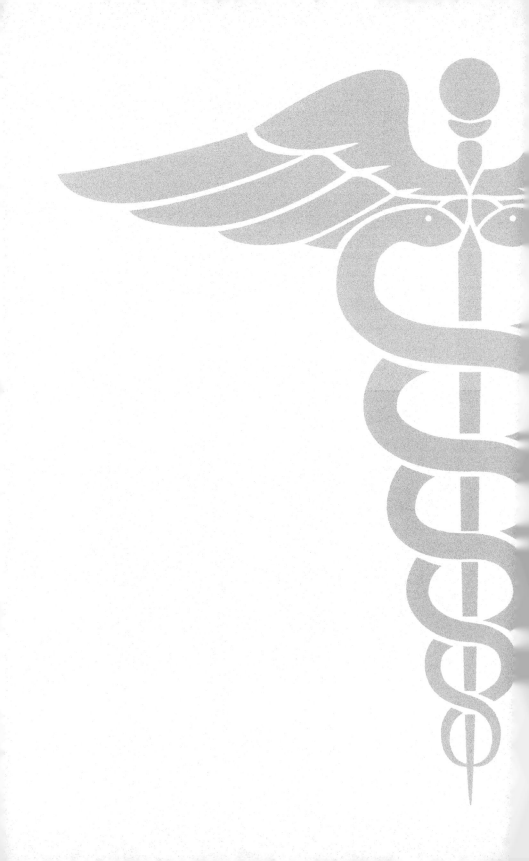

CHAPTER 7

Getting Old Beats the Alternative? 12:58 a.m.

"Doc, Kyle and Jason brought in a guy from the nursing home. Here's the chart," Dave reports as he hands me the clipboard for Room 5. CC: fever and shaking 81 y.o. male

I enter Room 5 and see a wrinkly faced man with scattered white wisps of hair failing to cover his balding head. His ocean blue eyes show a spacey look of confusion that might be from infection or baseline dementia. Surprisingly, his physique is solid and not the usual frail appearance that most nursing home patients have. He was probably an athlete back in his youth. In fact, his looks strike a memory that I have seen him or someone who looks just like him, before. Kyle is at the bedside, surprisingly assisting Nurse Dave. They are undressing the elderly patient and putting him in a gown. I don't ever remember Kyle helping in the routine nursing duties.

"Doc, old dude here was having rigors when I got the IV. I bet he is septic. Jason is cleaning the rig as senile dude pissed all over everything," Kyle chimes in. Kyle solved the two mysteries. My patient's probable diagnosis, and secondly, why he is helping Dave. For a paramedic, Kyle has a bad aversion to bodily fluid urine. "Oh, Doc, should I call Brandy to draw lab and blood cultures, please?" Kyle asks. I was mistaken again. Kyle was totally smitten by our night shift phlebotomist. He knew that this patient would need lab draws, including two blood cultures. He has badly wanted to ask out Brandy for weeks now. Each time he was close, he lost the nerve, or had an ambulance call. I couldn't blame him for wanting to ask her out or failing to act. Brandy was simply gorgeous. She had long, silky, black hair, and darker middle- eastern complexion with stunning features. She always wore a smile while carrying out her duties, which she did with speed and efficiency. A blood drawing wonder woman. If Gal Gadot worked as a phlebotomist/lab technician instead of an actress, you would have Brandy's older twin. I often felt bad for Brandy. Not that she had guys ogling her all the time, but for her actual job. In fact, not only her, but all her fellow lab colleagues. The role of lab technician is a vital, yet thankless job in the hospital. Often they are called to draw blood in the ED, then take those samples back to the hospital lab and process them. When they do their job well, the ED staff, me included, never acknowledge them. However, if they are slow or make any error, we are unforgiving. Something the staff and I should improve upon.

"Yes Kyle, call that sexy vampire of your dreams. Hell, if you want, I'll tell her you want to take her out for coffee in the morning," I offer.

"Yes, please Doc," Kyle responds. As I have mentioned before, it is good to keep your staff happy. Also, when Brandy enters the ED, Kyle becomes worthless. He loses focus and makes excuses to visit whatever patient from whom she happens to be drawing blood.

"Kyle, I'll help with Brandy. Now tell me as much as you can about our older, probably bacteremic patient here," I ask as I start to do my phys-ical exam on my new patient.

"Well, Doc he is a walkie non talkie. Nursing home said pretty demented, sometimes knows his name and makes purposeful gestures.

Spiked a fever and was incontinent with urine all day. He was shaking in the rig and temp was 102 degrees. He is a "full code" and the nursing home said daughter should be coming in later tonight," Kyle wraps up. The term "full code" is very important not only when taking care of patients in the ER, but with being a living human on the planet Earth. When someone is a full code, it means that everything possible will be done to save their life: Cardiopulmonary resuscitation (CPR), which includes chest compressions, intubation, and defibrillation. The other end of the spectrum is comfort measures only. This is when a person is both a DNR (Do Not Resuscitate, meaning no CPR) and in addition, doesn't want anything except treatment that can provide relief from any suffering. There are many options that a patient or family member can choose for their loved one that fall in between those two ends of the spectrum.

My older gentleman has his eyes wide open and is breathing rapidly. I push on his abdomen and don't get any response. Surprisingly, he does obey a few commands. When I listen to his lungs, he takes deep breaths at my request. Also, he moves his extremities well, but only when asked. The lights upstairs were on in his sparsely covered head. I am not sure how bright those lights usually radiate until his daughter shows up and informs me of his baseline. Elderly patients with fevers can become so confused that they can resemble a person in late stage Alzheimer's. Or, the infectious process with a normal temperature can still result in a delirium. I look up at the monitor and see his blood pressure is a bit low, 95 systolic over 45 diastolic. I need to be aggressive on his treatment and start pushing fluids. I quickly write orders that cover septic workup and treatment: cbc (complete blood count), comprehensive metabolic panel, lactic acid, urinalysis (UA), 2 blood cultures, chest x-ray, and IV bolus NS 2 liters, foley catheter placement, IV antibiotic Rocephin (start after blood cultures obtained), 1 gram Tylenol. A couple of tests that would be added today were not needed back then. Influenza season was well past and we rarely see cases in May. Likewise, the dreaded Covid virus was over a decade away from rearing its ugly head.

Let me share some information on feverish patients. A viral illness is the most common cause of any person's rising temperature. Hands down, viruses are the undisputed hard-hitting champion of fevers. Often, these are self-limiting, meaning over time it runs its course and you are back to normal after a week of feeling lousy. Don't we possess treatment for viruses? Sure, we physicians are armed with antiviral medication. Why are those medications not used more often? In most cases, the viruses are not deadly and in the few that are, we probably don't have a specific antiviral medicine to treat those. There are a few exceptions (HIV, Herpes, etc.) and medicines are being developed to treat viruses more than ever before, but the bacteria is the true king and queen of inflicting what I call, treatable infectious death. Putting trauma patients aside for the moment, how does the ED staff usually save lives? By far and away, the two things we give that save the most lives on any particular day in the ED are fluids and antibiotics in IV administration. Thus, our work up focuses on the possible bacterial source that we have medicine with which to treat it. The majority of elderly fever caused by bacteria usually comes down to three main sources: the lung, the skin, and what I am already guessing is my nonverbal old man's cause, the urine. Yes, there are many other bacterial causes, some of which include: sinusitis, meningitis, dental abscess, colitis, appendicitis, and cholecystitis (which is a gallbladder infection). However, when dealing with a common problem, look for the most common conclusion. Listen to the lungs and get a chest X-ray to assess for possible pneumonia. A quick visual exam of a patient's skin surface can quickly find or rule out a cellulitis, also known as a skin infection. Lastly, obtain or retrieve a urine specimen to look for the all-too-common urinary tract or bladder infection. Also, I want to point out, my elderly patient received the anti-biotic, Rocephin. It is a broad-spectrum antibiotic. This means it has the ability to treat many different types of bacteria. Our three big offenders most often come from three different bacteria. Pneumonia's number one is Streptococcus Pneumoniae. Most cellulitis is by far caused by Methicillin Resistant Staph Aureus (MRSA). Finally, Escherichia Coli (E. Coli) is the number one most wanted urine infector. Rocephin is an excellent first choice for both pneumonia and UTI, and not a bad start for cellulitis. Now, let's get back to our story of the elderly male with a presumed serious urinary infection.

I tell Dave my orders and give Kyle my clipboard so he can take it to Cindy. In seconds, Cindy will type my orders into her computer. A few minutes later I'm walking out of the room when Brandy walks in. I stop to turn back around. Brandy gives Dave and I one of her large, beaming smiles. It's easy to understand why Kyle is enamored by this bloodsucker. Remember, Brandy is a phlebotomist. She draws blood for a profession, aka bloodsucker. "Brandy, our patient here is confused, but seems to be pretty gentle. Kyle brought him in and gave me a great update on this fever-ish man," I offer. Brandy mouths a thank you and ties a small rubber tour-niquet to the patient's arm and preps the location for her blood draw. I wait until she inserts the needle and blood starts flowing into the first of many test tubes. I stand on the opposite side of the bed from Brandy and begin, "Brandy, I know it's not the perfect time, but because I know you can per-form your job blindfolded, I have a question for you." She looks up and is able to continue filling tubes and replacing a filled one with a new empty one while never taking her eyes off me. "Kyle really wants to go out with you. Do you have any interest in my stellar paramedic?"

Her smile gets even more alluring. I didn't think it was possible. "Of course I do. I get anxious every time I get paged to come down to the ED in hopes of running into him," Brandy answers. Well, looks like it's time to make Kyle's night.

"He gets done at 7AM. Your shift ends at 8, right?" She nods again. "Great, he'll grab you for coffee if that sounds good to you?" concluding my matchmaker mission.

"Yes, tell him I'm looking forward to it," Brandy confirms. I look over at Dave who appears a bit jealous, but who I know is happily married. As I walk out of the room, I turn to my nurse, "Dave if you need help with the foley, tell Kyle I said he can lend a hand." If you don't recall, Kyle doesn't like urine in the least. Worse than urine for Kyle though is handling an old man's penis. That act alone nearly gives Kyle a seizure. Of course, the placement of a foley is rather straightforward, if you aren't the patient that is. It is simply a flexible tube that is placed in the urethra through the penis opening in order to drain urine out of the bladder. What is important to know is how it stays attached to the body. There is a balloon port that 10 ccs of sterile water is injected into that inflates the balloon inside the bladder. The expanded balloon enables the catheter tip to not slip back out. Occasionally, patients who don't know about the balloon or who are confused yank the tube out without deflating the balloon. This causes trauma to the urethra and lots of bloody urine. I wouldn't force Kyle to do what he hates, but I only want to remind him that he now owes me for my assistance in setting him up with Brandy. Of course, I should call us even, after all the barrage of teasing I have put lonely Kyle through. The truth is, I have been relentlessly teasing him about his lack of action. He likes to talk a big talk and then when cupid's arrow finally hits him, he freezes. I have to admit his sloth-like motion in the love area has blessed me with ample ammunition to bring much needed humor to our sometimes depressing shifts. The idea of humor and the image of the patient's white wisps of hair give me a wave of nostalgia.

My memory is jolted back to residency and why this elderly patient looks so familiar. He looks identical to my famous Dr. Kramer patient. Technically he wasn't Dr. Kramer's actual patient, which was part of the reason it was so hilarious. I probably shouldn't tell this story because it may make us doctors appear to be monsters. Hell, we are human, for better or worse. Like all humans, we find coping mechanisms to get through tough days. The tv show MASH is a perfect example of physicians using humor to cope. In the fictional show, the surgeons Hawkeye Pierce and B.J. Hunnicutt joked their way through medical stress and war. Well, in my residency, Dr. Kramer was the real-life physician playing Alan Alda's Hawkeye to Dr. Peterson's playing the role of Hunnicutt. Both Doctors Peterson and Kramer were my senior residents. They had experienced a little more and knew slightly more than me. Eventually, with hard work and time, I would become their equal in treating patients. However, there was one area of expertise where my skills would never come close. That was their relentless practical joking. Kramer was more consistent and able to pull them off on a daily basis without much thought or setup. Peterson was usually methodical and planned his out. He played far fewer jokes on Kramer, but they were more lasting.

Before we get to Peterson's all-time best, let's discuss a typical Dr. Kramer joke. One of my personal favorite Kramer jokes utilized his spur of the moment style. Dr. Kramer liked to keep people on their toes and spice it up. He always had his ears open for the latest gossip, especially when that gossip entailed who was hooking up with who. If a new resident was fooling around with a nurse or two, Kramer made it his business to find out. He knew if the lab technician was dating the X-ray technician. When the hot ED secretary got engaged, Kramer knew when her last two flings ended and that the third fling was still secretly going on. He used this type of information to burn Dr. Peterson on a few occasions.

I arrived for one particular shift and as usual Kramer wasn't taking a shift off. I was coming on as Kramer was leaving. I needed to see if he had any patients to hand off. I walked around the ED looking for Dr. Kramer when suddenly I heard, "DOCTOR! DOCTOR! We need a doctor in the bathroom near exam room 8. SOMEONE HEARD A FALL! THEY'RE NOT BREATHING. HELP! HELP!" Well, the someone yelling from behind an exam room curtain was Dr. Kramer, altering his voice. In the busy ED it is hard to identify even familiar voices. I recognized the voice because that was for whom I was searching, and I had peeked behind the curtain to see who was yelling for help. Five minutes earlier, Kramer had told every nurse to disregard the "soon-to-be call for 'help'" in the bathroom. Kramer knew our smoking hot secretary was secretly seeing our attending physician, Dr. Greenly. What he also knew was Dr. Greenly and the secretary had snuck off to rendezvous in the bathroom by Room 8. That bathroom also had a faulty lock of which Dr. Kramer was aware. The lock mechanism would read "locked" when engaged, but no longer actually locked the door. As I headed for the bathroom, Kramer grabbed my arm and said, "Dude, no one fell, I'm trying to get Peterson." I looked around and didn't see our attending physician, but did see Dr. Peterson running to check on the supposedly sick and possibly dying patient in the bathroom by 8. I looked at Kramer and asked, "Who is in the bathroom?" All he did was grin mischievously and start laughing. I briskly walked over to witness Dr. Peterson yank the bathroom door wide open. Right behind me were four of the ED nurses, a lab tech, two ED techs, and standing behind everyone, Dr. Kramer, the mad conductor. The focus of everybody's eyes was the now open bathroom. Dr. Greenly had his scrub pants around his ankles and his bare white ass mooning the entire staff. The engaged secretary was bent over the sink, most of her naked body blocked from view, but not everything. Dr. Peterson now stood in front of the open door dumbfounded with no clue what to do. He slowly started to close the door when somebody yelled, "Dr. Peterson saved another one!" Of course, Dr. Kramer had to make sure everybody knew who had opened the door. Not only did Peterson open the door on his attending, but he was played like a fiddle by Kramer. (On a more serious note: hot secretary broke off her prior engagement and did eventually become Mrs. Dr. Greenly).

Peterson lost many battles, but the practical joke war raged on. My favorite of all time looked so similar to my elderly nonverbal feverish patient, they could have been twins separated at birth. I recall the similarly shaped, nearly bald head as it was yesterday. Even the similar muscular build for a man late in life and sadly demented. Yes, Peterson and Kramer used any means at their disposal. One would think a demented patient was off limits. Well, they would be wrong. I was working my shift along with Peterson when my doppelgänger patient presented. Like my current patient, he had fevers and shakes. I had diagnosed him as having urosepsis (urine infection that leads to serious full body illness) and began treatment, planning for admission. The only glaring difference between the two was this earlier residency patient was verbal. Not only was he verbal, but he also screamed every word that came out of his mouth. Early in my work up, I was assessing his cognition and saw his mouth resembled a desert. His oral mucosa was so dry it was flaking. I said to him, "would you like water?"

He responded, not saying, but yelling, "WATER! WATER! WATER! WATER! WATER! WATER! WATER!" He didn't stop until a cup of water reached his lips. I ordered the nurse to have one large container of water and another of juice at bedside and within reach at all times. His screams had scared half the patients in the ED. The other half thought it was funny. It isn't funny at all, but you know the old saying, "better to laugh than cry!" One of those who was laughing, and at the same time plotting with his devious mind, was Dr. Peterson. Unbeknownst to me, Dr. Peterson stealthily made his way into my megaphone talker's room. Peterson laid his groundwork for a devious practical joke. Dr. Kramer was due to start his shift in about an hour, exactly when Dr. Peterson's shift was ending. What I would later discover after grilling Peterson for information was how simple it was to set his heinous plan in motion. Peterson told my demented patient that I (Dr. Adams) was leaving, but that his new doctor, Dr. Kramer would be coming on soon. Peterson encouraged the patient to say, "DOCTOR KRAMER!" not only once, but repeatedly nonstop and never tire or waver in intensity. How exactly he managed to pull this off, he never divulged. When I first heard Dr. Kramer's name yelled, I was confused because Kramer wasn't due for an hour. Then it hit me. Peterson is messing with my patient. I ran over to the old screamer's room. Peterson was at bedside finishing his nefarious mission by telling my patient, "Doctor Kramer! Say, Doctor Kramer! again," Peterson continued and the patient yelled, "DOCTOR KRAMER! DOCTOR KRAMER!" Peterson was smiling and trying, but failing, to stifle his laughter.

I was initially pissed because this was my patient with whom he was messing. Even as a young resident, I took ownership of my patients and that responsibility seriously. Peterson was also my superior so I was conflicted. However, when I looked down at the screaming grandpa's face, he was smiling each time he finished yelling "DOCTOR KRAMER!" He actually looked to be enjoying himself. Peterson had convinced him that by yelling "Dr. Kramer," his wildest dreams would come true or something equivalent. It was true that one person's wish was coming true. Peterson had the biggest grin whenever the old guy yelled, "DOCTOR KRAMER!" The next ten minutes were non-stop ear piercing, "DOCTOR KRAMER! DOCTOR KRAMER! DOCTOR KRAMER!" over and over again. Nobody but Peterson was happy. It was so loud that nobody could think straight and the entire staff was getting irritable. I tried to get him to say water again. No luck. I tried other words, but he was convinced by yelling, "DOCTOR KRAMER," everything in the world would be right. I ended up sedating my patient, so the ED could function properly. Peterson begged me not to give him more than 30-40 minutes' worth of medication. He wanted to get the patient screaming "DOCTOR KRAMER!" when Kramer actually walked in to start his shift. I hoped the patient would not remember the name that had been planted in his brain. I reluctantly obliged my senior resident's request for a lower dosage of the sedation medication.

At five minutes to change of shift, Peterson actually went in and woke up my sleeping screamer. "Dr. Kramer's here and will be your doctor all night long. You remember Dr. Kramer?" Peterson prodded and some-how convinced the patient to perform right on cue. "DOCTOR KRAMER! DOCTOR KRAMER! DOCTOR KRAMER!" the yelling commenced. Headaches that had faded began anew. Newly arrived patients started asking who is this Dr. Kramer? They didn't want to see him if they had a choice in the matter. Most importantly, to Peterson anyway, Kramer walked into the ED completely stupefied. Kramer could hear his name being yelled the moment he got out of his car, as he approached for ER duty. Peterson told Kramer he had nobody to hand off except my banshee who was screaming his name. It wasn't his patient to hand off, but my headache forced me to go along. The night shift staff tried to get Mr. Scream up to his admitted hospital bed and out of the ED as quickly as possible, but it took hours. Kramer confided that he was so pissed hearing his name yelled out for half the night he vowed to make Peterson pay like never before.

If the story ended there it would have been amusing—a successfully played practical joke on a nemesis. The evil mastermind physician (Dr. Peterson) had chalked the screamer incident as a success. The ruckus produced by yelling Dr. Kramer's name and the pure volume of the patient's screaming proved his septic picture was in the rearview mirror. Successful I agree, but Peterson had no idea how big a success he had actually pulled off. Days later, I was heading for my first day of a month-long Intensive Care Unit (ICU) rotation. During residency we spend only half of our three years in the ED. We spend the rest of our time in multiple other fields including surgery, orthopedics, and radiology, along with elective rotations around the hospital or even out of state.

Anyway, I was walking up the stairs toward the ICU when I heard some yelling. "DOCTOR KRAMER! DOCTOR KRAMER! DOCTOR KRAMER!" projected down the stairwell. I will admit I started to cry. Not because I was sensitive and sad. No, I was laughing so bloody hard, tears were welling up in my eyes. It sounds terrible, but I couldn't help it. It had been four or five days since I had admitted Mr. Scream. He should have been well enough after three days of treatment to be discharged home. I wiped my eyes and bit my tongue as I went to investigate why he hadn't been discharged yet. The tongue biting is a technique I have employed to stop laughing at inappropriate times. Of course, the screaming became more intense the closer I got to the source.

The nearby nurses station was empty. I looked around the corner to the far end of that hospital wing and saw all the nurses for the entire floor huddled around one small distant station. I made the walk over as the piercing "DOCTOR KRAMER! DOCTOR KRAMER!" pleasantly lessened the further I went away from the source. My ear drums slowly stopped ringing. The nurses saw me coming and before I could ask why he hadn't been discharged, three of the nurses asked, "Do you know who this Dr. Kramer is?" They proceeded to inform me that he screamed "DOCTOR KRAMER!" all night and day and only stopped when one of the hospital doctors added sedation medicine. Every nurse had looked through Mr. Screamer's entire chart and Kramer's name wasn't anywhere to be found. The reason the floor nurses did not know who Dr. Kramer was, is that large teaching hospitals have over a hundred attending physicians. In addition, floor nurses would rarely know resident physicians from other departments. This lack of knowledge had put the nurses in a quandary. The family had refused to take our elderly patient home until Dr. Kramer came to see him or the screaming stopped. After the nurses explained the situation, I started laughing so hard, I nearly peed my pants. The nurses glared daggers at me and likely wanted to stab me. My one hour screaming onslaught in the ED was nothing. These poor nurses had to deal with multiple 12-hour shifts with "DOCTOR KRAMER!" ringing in their ears. Not to mention the suffering floor patients.

Ok, the madness needed to come to an end. I didn't cause it, but I also hadn't stopped it. Summoning all my strength and stuffing Kleenex in my ears, I was ready for the mission. The only analogy that I can offer is if you are familiar with the Marvel movie "Logan." I was walking toward a voice that was so shrill and loud it caused physical pain. My old patient had become more powerful with days of practice projecting his auditory vocal cannon. I was like Wolverine, having to use his healing superpowers to walk toward the mind blasting power of a demented Professor Xavier. Even with plugged ear canals, the eardrums felt like they were bleeding. It seemed to intensify the closer I came to the source. As I stepped toward "DOCTOR KRAMER! DOCTOR KRAMER!" I reached his bedside and my prior patient stopped his screaming. He had a flicker of recognition when he stared up at me. Exhaustion was written all over his face. He was about to start yelling again when I grabbed his hand and looked him in his eyes. I didn't replicate Peterson's voodoo magic, but talked calmly and gently like he was a child. "You remember me. You go home now. You don't need doctor. Doctors all gone. You all good. Home now," I finished with the most reassuring smile I could muster. He smiled back. Next thing I knew he was closing his eyes. He was snoring before I had time to leave the room. I walked out of that room like a champion. All the nurses who a few minutes ago wanted to kill me, now looked like they wanted to give me a kiss. Yes, we physicians can fix chaos. Pathetically, we can also be the hilarious cause of it as well.

Boring is something the ED staff crave after midnight. Thankfully, the next few patients were simple and unexciting: A one year old with an upper respiratory infection who mom brought in because he spiked a fever. Another was a teenage girl with a sore throat. Basically, the run of the mill Urgent Care after 1 AM crowd. Nevertheless, a dull ED rarely stays that way. Before things picked up, I had a window of opportunity. I eyed my stack of charts sitting on my desk. Early in the shift, I contemplated keeping up with them as the hours and patients went by. However, the volume of patients was too much for me to include charting. It rarely happens to me, but I gave up. I decided to wait for a long break between new patient arrivals. Sometimes that break never appears. What I really needed was an hour of no patients. If that happened, I could start dictating and document my patient encounters and actually do charting. The dreaded alternative is to stay after the shift is over and work longer. Yippee, sign me up for that shit. Unfortunately, it happens so much now in medicine, it has become normal. Work your butt off so much that when your shift is over, the least fun work begins. Right when you're all done and it's time to go home, nope not yet. The more you desire that post shift drink, the longer you'll be waiting to get it.

Anyway, sorry for the whining, let's continue. As soon as I can discharge my two simple patients, then maybe I can focus on the charting. I type up the two discharges but before I can hand them to a nurse, I hear a commotion break out. As is always the case with the quiet ED, something or someone breaks the silence. Suddenly, I see the cause of the ruckus. I am sitting at my desk and my demented nonverbal patient is staggering in the hallway corridor. Somehow, he had maneuvered himself off the exam bed that had both side railings locked in the raised position. As disconcerting as the stumbling is, there is a striking aspect to the picture that is much worse. He is totally naked. His pale wrinkled body is floundering like a baby deer trying to find his balance after being born. There is one final cringe worthy detail to put the final touches on the scene. The foley catheter is still hanging out of his penis. The catheter's attached collection bag is behind, being dragged along the ground.

As my naked scared patient teeters back and forth for stability, someone yells "Ahhh!" I turned and see it is the mother of the feverish baby yelling.

"Oh my God!" the teenager says, likely forgetting about her sore throat. I stand up slowly from my desk and gingerly make my way toward my naked, demented, foley-dangling patient. Moving quickly or aggressively could startle him and chances are a fall would only exacerbate the situation. We don't need any additional problems added to this already worrisome spectacle.

As Nurse Sharon approaches from his right, I came along on his left. Before either of us reached him, his wobbly legs stabilize. It is miraculous. With his new found strength, his pace quickens and he zips past Sharon and I. This reassures me that he is less likely to fall, but now I am worried he will be harder to catch. I was also worried that the foley catheter dragging behind him will catch on something and be ripped out. I quickly sprint to get back in front of him, so I can reassure him as I secure him.

"Grab him!" somebody yells. From my new position, I witness a scary new expression appear on his prior confused face. He now wore a psychotic smile that reminds me of Batman's joker. The sides of his smile seem to be unnaturally elevated. Of course, the patients and their family members created an ED audience that contributed to instill terror in my naked foley dragger. The terror must have boosted his adrenalin and given him energy along with the IV fluids he recently received. I notice the foley catheter that was half filled with urine is now slowly turning red. The weight of the urine in the dragging foley bag is causing trauma.

Just as I notice the blood draining from the foley tube, my patient looks down at his penis. Oh no, he is going to yank out his foley. This would result in him running around the ED dripping blood from his damaged member. Obviously, that would be a step in the wrong direction. I notice Kyle peek around a nearby corner, then slowly disappear back the direction he had come. Kyle had seen the focus of the ED's attention and this was the only type of drama he wanted nothing to do with. Now that it was taking longer to corral my runaway, I figure his body would fatigue enough to bring an easy end to his adventure. I was soon proven wrong. Not only did he not tire, but he also found some extra energy. Remember when he noticed his penis with a tube hanging out of it? Well, his eyes followed that tube to the trailing collecting urine filled bag. Instead of pulling the tube out as I feared, he picked up the bag and tucked it under his right arm. He is now carrying the foley bag like it was a football and he was the star running back. Once the bag is secured in the right arm crook, his speed amplifies. Nurses Dave and Judy try to cut him off and he side-steps both of them. After escaping the double team, he has an open field and his prior psychotic smile turns to one of gleeful joy. He was enjoying himself as he is rushing down the back hall of the ED.

Melody was coming back from a break and with her pregnant belly wasn't in great tackling condition. She steps back toward the wall, leaving the closed back door exposed. However, the back door uses an ID lock, so only staff can open it with their key cards. Foley streaker is trapped. When he reaches the locked door, he pivots to turn and face me and the rest of the staff. It almost looks like he was posing for us. He didn't, but I like to imagine him extending his left arm in a stiff-arm motion while lifting left knee up and pulling off the Heisman pose. What he does is actually more memorable. He runs right at us, daring us to tackle him, like a game of high stakes chicken. As he builds up speed and shortens the distance to us, I tell the staff, "Let him run! Steer clear if you can." He is having fun and I think is ready to inflict damage on any would-be tacklers. We all step out of the way as he actually runs past us back toward his room. He stops, and I am worried he might spike the foley like he had scored a touchdown. Instead, he slows down and points with his left hand to his now empty bed. Extreme exhaustion has caught up with him. He flops down on the end of the bed still gripping the foley football. As the nurses maneuver him further into bed and cover him up with a sheet, something totally dawns on me. Holy shit, his daughter is due to enter the ED any minute now. She could have arrived at any time when he was running buck naked with a foley dangling from his penis all around the ED. She would have been mortified. "Doc, he won't let go of the foley bag," Dave informs me. I step to the head of the bed and put my hand on his right arm. He squeezes the foley bag dangerously tight.

"You scored the game winning touchdown, game over. I'll hook your football foley to the bed rail. Ok?" I beg him. His lips form a smile as he loosens his grip. I reach for the foley bag.

"What about a game winning touchdown?" a voice from behind me asks. I look back and standing in the doorway is a classy dressed middle-aged woman. "That's my father. Are you the doctor?" she asks.

I nonchalantly hook the foley bag to the bed rail, then introduce myself. "Yes, I'm Dr. Adams. Was your father a football player in his youth?"

She is slightly stunned by my question then responds, "He was a star running back in high school and even got a college scholarship back in the day. Why do you ask?"

I need to tread carefully. No way was I going to tell this elegantly dressed woman her dad scampered nude around the ED for the past 10 minutes.

"Um, well he is more muscular than most men in their eighties. I figured he had to be an athlete." I hope she buys it.

"With his dementia so severe these days, the only time he seems to show any emotion is when a football game is on tv. His eyes open wider and sometimes we see him smile when the running back makes a big play," she confides.

Crisis averted! Thankfully, no evidence exists because the first iPhones were in their infancy and nobody had recorded my naked foley carrying running back dashing around the ED.

Later that night, Dave and Judy asked me why I let the naked patient run around for so long. I gave them a quick explanation about it might be his last opportunity for an enjoyable experience in his life. *I won't take that away.* I didn't tell them I actually consider the patient's end of life pleasure a part of my responsibility as a physician. We are trained to limit pain and suffering. But why stop at simply limiting pain and discomfort? When I might have the opportunity to give someone their final wish, I won't ever deny that.

Years before I became a doctor, I learned a valuable lesson from a physician's mistake. I was starting my third year of medical school and doing rotations in the hospital. It was really the first time I was experiencing direct hands-on patient encounters. Most medical training consists of two years of book work. We used to call it our didactic years. We have many class lectures, lab time including hands on cadavers for anatomy, and on the rare occasion do a hospital or clinic day seeing real patients. Starting our third year we leave the lecture halls for the hospital. We start shadowing physicians on a more consistent basis. That was when I learned making someone happy can be more important than keeping someone alive. I was shadowing an internal medicine doctor or internist (Dr. Clark). He had a clinic and also saw patients in the hospital. These days that is a rarity. Most doctors will work in a clinic or hospital, rarely both. He had me print out his patient list each morning and visit every one of his hospital patients before he arrived each day. I would check their most recent lab and vitals, compare it to prior days, and talk to the patients. I was still two years away from the title of "Doctor," so when I conversed with patients it was like a normal person would talk to you, not like a medical professional. Of course I asked them how they felt, but also what they were looking forward to when they left the hospital. I remember one elderly gentleman's face well, but can't recall his name. Let's call him Frank. He was hospitalized for congestive heart failure (CHF) after suffering a major heart attack. He had undergone a cardiac catheterization but no intervention was warranted. In all honesty, he was lucky to still be alive and most of his doctors were convinced he wouldn't survive to discharge. His main treatable problem was the CHF, which is when fluid builds up in the lungs and compromises breathing. The main treatment is to decrease the fluid in the body by optimizing the heart's ability and by simply urinating a lot. To increase urine, we use diuresis medications called diuretics. We also limit the intake of oral fluids. Each day we measure patients weight along with how much fluid they ingest and how much they expel. We term it "I's and O's," for ins and outs. Frank had been put on a strict limit of oral intake and we were making him pee around the clock. His breathing continued to show minuscule improvement each day and his weight edged lower. With his continued improvement, he was due to go home soon. We couldn't do much more for him in the hospital. Truth was, his cardiac function was dangerously low and any day really could be his last. We had optimized his medical care and there wasn't much more we could do.

One morning after checking labs, I's, O's, and vitals, I walked into Frank's room. Everything was looking fine and Frank was progressing as well as could be expected. "Morning Frank, how are you feeling today?" I asked.

"Hi student doctor, doing great except thirsty," Frank responded. He liked calling me "student doctor after I had explained to him I wore the shorter white lab coat because I was still a medical student and not yet a doctor. "Student doc, I am craving a beer more than anything. Do you think Dr. Clark will let me increase my fluid intake a little?" Frank asked.

"No promises Frank, but I'll ask him. If you tell him how badly you want one, that will help your cause," I replied.

An hour later I walked back into Frank's room. This time I was accompanied by Dr. Clark. "Hi Frank, I heard you might be good enough for discharge in the morning. I also heard you were lusting for a beer," Dr. Clark stated.

Frank looked over at me. He looked pleasantly surprised that I had relayed his request. "Yeah Doc. If I could have one beer tonight, I won't drink anything else, I promise," Frank begged. I looked at Dr. Clark's face as he contemplated his patient's request. I also looked at Frank and saw the hope in his eyes as he was picturing a cold beer in his hand.

After what felt like a few minutes but was probably seconds, Dr. Clark made his decision, "Frank, tomorrow if you continue to improve I'll discharge you and you can have a beer when you get home." I could see Frank's face fall in disappointment as he heard Dr. Clark's words. I felt bad for Frank and didn't see the harm one beer would cause. As we walked to the next patient's room Dr. Clark told me he almost honored Frank's request. The reason he didn't was he didn't want to set a precedent on allowing one of his patient's to bring in and consume alcohol in the hospital.

The next morning as I printed off Dr. Clark's patient list I was thinking how happy Frank would be knowing he might soon be home drinking a beer. As you have already guessed, Frank's name was not on the list. Frank had died in his sleep sometime in the middle of the night. Damn it. I was pissed and actually confused. Where was this anger really coming from though? After thinking about it, I realized I wasn't mad or sad that Frank died. He was probably going to die any day and going in your sleep is really the best death one can get. I was angry that Dr. Clark hadn't let him have that beer. Why keep living if there is no pleasure? Frank's answer was, we don't. His heart attack had been massive and after surviving, he only wanted one thing. That one thing was denied so he stopped fighting and his body gave up. Of course, it wasn't that straight forward, but my mind focused on that one thing Frank desired—the beer. When Dr. Clark came in an hour later he was very gloomy. He told me, "Wow, I got the call about Frank at 2AM and wasn't able to get back to sleep. I'm kicking myself that

I didn't allow him to have that damn beer." Dr. Clark looked me in the eye and said, "Learn from my mistake so something positive can come from my poor decision."

I immediately felt guilty for having been angry at Dr. Clark and told him, "In those few days, Frank made an impression on me and if it's in my power I'll remember to honor my future patient's last wishes." Turning back to my demented, nonverbal, naked, foley swinging, former football playing patient, well, he couldn't tell me what his final wish was, but I granted him one I think he enjoyed. (I followed the hospital course of my football foley patient. He never ambulated again without using a walker and died a month later in the rehab area of the hospital, never making it home).

I sit back down at my desk once again eyeing the large stack of charts. I am about to pick the top one up when, "BEEP! BEEP! BEEP!" The EMS radio goes off with a police notification. "This is Officer Charles on the way to the hospital! I am escorting an elderly gentleman with huge tongue swelling! Be there in four to five minutes, officer out!"

Nurse Sharon is near the radio. She picked up the intercom and replies, "This is ER, message received, see you in four minutes, ER clear!"

Well, so much for considering those stinking charts. "Prep Room 2 and bring the crash cart and airway cart," I instruct. EDs have various carts for particular issues. The crash cart is for pulseless, non-breathing patients who come in with CPR in progress. The airway cart is self-explanatory. What is inside the airway cart might not be. We have the endotracheal tubes in addition to cricothyroidotomy (CTT) kits. The CTT kit enables fatal obstructions to become open airways. Far from what is shown on tv and film, we don't do tracheostomies in the ED. Those are done in the OR. They are bloody and longer procedures than the surprisingly simple CTT.

I hear the police siren approaching and make my way to the ambulance doors. A police car rolls through and stops a car length past the entrance. An old Cadillac stops behind the police car, right in front of the doors and the driver steps out. He is a gray-haired man moving slowly but deliberately. This man has to be over eighty years old, I surmise. I walk toward him as he points to his massively protruding tongue. His tongue is so swollen it extends inches out of his mouth, separating his upper and lower lips farther apart than I thought humanly possible. He has oral angioedema. This is swelling under the skin and is life threatening when it occurs near one's airway. His condition is serious as airway compromise might be imminent, I have no idea if swelling is occurring elsewhere in the airway anatomy. He hands me his driver's license. I look down at his name. "Follow me Mr. Jackson. I'm Dr. Adams. Do you take blood pressure medicine?" I ask. He nods. I must rely on his head movement. There is no way he's talking with that gigantic tongue of his. We help him to the exam bed and raise the head of the bed up to a 90-degree angle. He is sitting up right as I start rattling off a bunch of names from the ace inhibitor type of blood pressure medications. It is rare, but ace inhibitors are the leading cause of drug induced angioedema. He nods to one of the names I stated. It isn't common, but the drug group is so prevalently used that I have seen severe angioedema from ace inhibitors at least a couple times every year. I tell Nurse Dave to push IV Solu-Medrol, Benadryl and Epinephrine. Also, to start an Epinephrine drip. As back up, I pull out the CTT kit and place it next to his bed. If he has no improvement with medication, I'm going to open a hole in his throat and place a tube so he can breathe.

My patient gets my attention and starts to imitate a painter. He is drawing in the air and then I realize I have to start playing charades. He isn't painting, he wants a pen and paper to tell me something. I get him a pen and paper as Dave is speedily pushing the IV medications. He starts writing frantically. The police officer peeks his head in and says, "Doc, this bloke has an emergency right? I shouldn't give him a ticket for speeding?"

I see my patient continue writing as I respond to the officer, "Oh, yes he has a true emergency. He isn't out of the woods yet. I would advise against a ticket, Officer."

The officer states, "I thought so. He was going over 60 mph in the 30 zone when I pulled him over. I walked over to his window and he pointed at his tongue. He started mumbling what I thought sounded like ER. So, I told him to follow me and we went over 80 mph for the last five miles here." I listen intently to the officer's story of this poor swollen guy keeping his cool under panicky conditions. Surprisingly, he seems more nervous now that he made it to the ED.

"Thanks Officer, you did great. I'll take it from here," I respond. Mr. Jackson hands me the paper he was writing on. The scribbly penmanship read the following, "Wife on toilet home. She has MS stuck toilet need help. Took her bathroom when tongue swell woke me. Got worse, she say go ER leave her. Please help wife!"

I suddenly picture a frail older woman sitting on a toilet worried sick about her husband's tongue expanding. She has no idea that he made it to the ED. In her mind, his airway could have closed causing him to drive his car off the road. Hell, she is probably picturing her husband dead in a ditch. I have to get this lady help as well. "Officer Charles!" I yell after reading the note. The officer had made it halfway to his squad car and heard me yell. He turns around and walks back. I hand him the note and after reading it, he goes and tells my patient, "I'll go help your wife, no problem. Give me his license, I'll leave right now to get her off that toilet," Officer Charles reassures us. Mr. Jackson then leans back into the bed. His shoulders slump and the rest of his body relaxes, knowing his wife would be taken care of.

He was relaxed, but my sphincter wasn't. I was still very worried about his airway. A month ago, I had another angioedema of the tongue patient who didn't respond to medication. I had to intubate him as his tongue continued to swell even after IV treatment was initiated. There is no way I would be able to intubate Mr. Jackson. The medication needs to work or I will have to create a surgical airway. When my prior patient had arrived, his tongue was double its normal size, not twenty times the size, like Mr. Jackson's. Unfortunately, that last tongue swelling patient's tongue doubled while in the ED. What was fortunate, he actually let me do a non-sedation intubation. I gave him no IV medications, only using a numbing spray on the back of his throat. I then placed the endotracheal tube down while he was completely conscious. It went smoothly, and once the airway was secure, I gave him sedation medicine. The worry with sedating these patients is they may stop breathing and establishing an airway becomes a race against time. With a compromised airway, you have less time with the most difficult cases. In Mr. Jackson's case, intubation wasn't an option. If medication didn't work, I would be slicing a new airway. I needed to keep an eye on the clock. "Dave, how many minutes since you gave the medications?"

"Only been four minutes, Doc." I need to stay calm and give the meds a few more minutes. However, I need to be ready to act if I see him laboring for air. "Mr. Jackson, does it feel swollen deep in your throat?" He shakes his head side to side. "Great, only feel that tongue is swollen?" He nods up and down again. "Ok, we have some time for the medicine to work. Do you feel any difference since the medicine was given?" He nods again. "Better?" He continued to nod and my sphincter started to relax as well. While I was asking him questions, his tongue started to slowly decrease in size. "Yes, I think it is getting smaller! Dave, what is your opinion?" I ask.

"I agree, Doc." I let out a sigh of relief as every procedure can have consequences, but a mistake establishing an airway has a higher chance of leaving you with a dead patient than other procedures. An hour later, Mr. Jackson was actually able to close his mouth. He was admitted to the ICU and discharged 24 hours later. Officer Charles rescued the wife off the toilet and reassured her that her husband was well.

My elderly tongue swelling patient remained calm and cognizant his entire hospital course. At over eighty years old, his memory was as sharp as a tack. Many elderly, like my foley and Dr. Kramer patient, weren't so lucky. Medical providers are reminded daily about our own mortality. However, as sad as the idea of death is, it is a part of life. What I find more frightening is what state of being we may find ourselves or our loved ones in as we journey toward that end. Losing one's mind from dementia tops that list. Dementia from Alzheimer's, Lewy body, vascular or other, I would argue is human's most feared disease process.

I hate dwelling on such a negative, so let's turn my frown upside down and make a little lemonade. I want to share with you a personal embarrassing story that I have shared with others that brought laughter in the face of my discomfort.

During my last year of medical school, I spent a weekend at my girlfriend's house. It was going to be my first time meeting her parents. We had been together for over two years and meeting her parents was the obvious next step. My girlfriend informed me that her grandmother would also be spending the weekend. Unfortunately, her mom's mother had recently been diagnosed with Alzheimer's. They had to take away her car keys and move her into an assisted living facility. The initial meeting went smoothly and we had a wonderful dinner. Her parents were easy to talk with and we got along well. The grandmother sat mute all through dinner. After dinner was finished, my girlfriend's father excused himself and went downstairs to read the newspaper. I stayed at the table to make conversation. The grandmother remained silent following dinner, but seemed to be staring more intently at me, and then occasionally would switch to stare at her granddaughter, my girlfriend, and future wife. I was starting to feel a little uncomfortable by how intense Grandma continued to stare at me. Before I could excuse myself, the grandmother stared directly at me and said her first words of the entire evening. "DO YOU TWO FUCK?" Everybody except the grandmother became speechless. She continued asking the question. I stammered and excused myself. I walked downstairs and my future father-in-law, who had been listening, asked me, "So what's the answer to the question?" I froze again and was considering how to respond when he countered with, "I'm messing with you. You don't have to answer, but remember, no matter how old they get, always fear the mother-in-law."

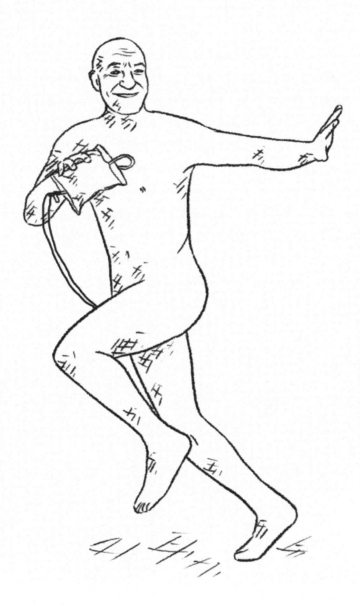

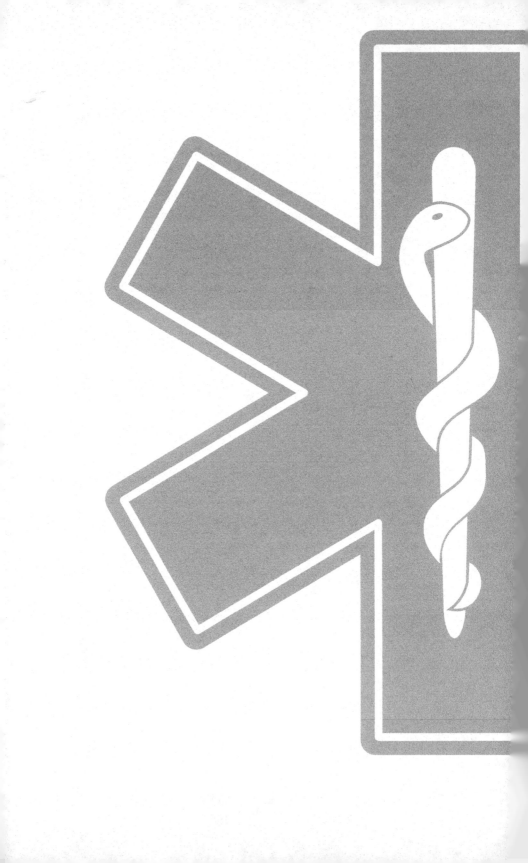

CHAPTER 8

What the F***? 2:14 a.m.

"BEEP! BEEP! BEEP!" "Police officer calling for EMS assist at Bay Hotel parking lot. An unresponsive young male found in a parked van."

"See you guys soon! After we give the Narcan, he'll probably bolt," Jason says as he and Kyle rush out the ambulance bay doors. Jason was referring to the now well-known antidote for opioid overdose. This case occurred back before Wave Two of the opioid epidemic. Narcan, (generic Naloxone) wasn't yet a household name. According to the U.S. Centers for Disease Control and Prevention (CDC), the United States has had three waves of the opioid epidemic. Wave One was during the 90's when pre-scription opioids were starting their rise. Wave Two began in 2010 when heroin became a more prolific addition to the overdose party, and finally in 2013 Fentanyl became the new, even more deadly member of the gang. Last year over 100,000 drug overdose deaths occurred in America. Opiates make up a majority of that staggering count. What is equally amazing, Narcan kits now in public hands saved 27,000 lives last year from adding to that number. Most paramedics are now pretty cynical when they hear a young person is found down. Every call that deals with a non-traumatic young unresponsive patient, paramedics figure it has to be a drug overdose.

The Bay Hotel is close, so they should arrive there quickly. After accessing and rendering emergency treatment, if needed, the medics will give me and the staff a report. I might have time to knock off a few charts. The problem is getting interrupted if I'm in dictation mode. I decide that I'll ease up and do nothing for ten minutes and take a much-needed breather. By "nothing," I refer to no medical duties. I motor to the back break-room, and grab a snack and drink some water. Sometimes it is in one's best interest to leave the damn charts until the shift is finished.

"BEEP! BEEP! BEEP!" "Medic 1 coming in with a 30ish male patient unresponsive but breathing. No change with Narcan. Possible seizure, now post ictal. Vitals stable! be there in five, medic 1 out!"

Judy responds to the EMS call, "ER copies, see you in five, ER clear!"

I say to anyone within hearing distance, "I love when we have butt breathers!" None of my staff laugh. "Come on guys, lighten up," I urge. I had a few paramedics who always teased their colleagues when they'd say "but breathing!" as part of the report over the radio. I found the bathroom humor kind of funny. Truthfully, I am actually happy he was "butt breathing," as it meant the transporting patient was not likely dying. However, he said the patient had no response to Narcan and possibly had a seizure. Sounds like this case won't be the straight forward opiate overdose as initially expected.

The ambulance pulls up with a police car right behind. On the gurney was a young male in his late twenties or early thirties wearing a plain white t-shirt and blue jeans. He looks like he was sleeping comfortably. He has a lot of facial hair scruff indicating that he hasn't shaved in a while. "Bring him to Room 6," Nurse Sharon instructs. I palpated his pulse on his wrist as we wheel the bed to Room 6. The pulse is strong, regular, and had a normal rate. A medical normal rate is 60 to 100. Below 60 is termed Bradycardia, or slow heart rate. Over 100 is Tachycardia or fast heart rate. Of course, many people's normal may fall outside that range. I know some extreme endurance athletes who have resting rates in the upper 30's. Likewise, I've treated chronic cardiac patients that live with heart rates at 100 even with rate lowering medication. My new patient's rate was about 65 and I would know his current blood pressure soon. Dave hooked him up to the monitor as Sharon accessed the paramedic's IV and then connected a liter of fluid to it. Blood pressure was 120/60. Basically, a perfect BP.

"Doc, he hasn't budged the entire time. Never flinched when I did a sternal rub or started the IV. We even did smelling salts. Doc, you need to talk to the police officer," Kyle tells me.

Walking into the room, as Kyle alluded to, is the police officer. She is a fit looking, short black woman about my age. She carries herself like a woman who doesn't put up with nonsense. Her brown piercing eyes look up to me as she asks, "Are you the doctor? I'm Officer James. Kinda ironic that I ended up in the ER anyway. At the start of my shift, I was heading this way when they said they no longer needed me here. Instead, I was diverted to a possible pervert in a van." This would have been my cavity searcher for my cocaine stuffer.

Even with her small stature, the blue police uniform and belt over-flowing with tactical gear, she has me intimidated. "Yes, I'm Dr. Adams. What else can you tell me about this guy?"

Her eyes seem to gain intensity as she recalls the incident. "Well, I got a call about a dude in a van staring at the prom kids swimming at the Bay Hotel. The pool is on the first floor and has large windows, so some areas of the parking lot look right in. The hotel has what seems like half the school staying there and they kept the pool open all night. Our fellow seemed to be gawking at the girls in their bikinis. I pulled my squad car up and he didn't notice me. I got out and walked to the driver side of his van. The dude was masturbating. He was jerking off while ogling at the girls. I knocked on the van door and he started seizing. I then called the ambulance and he didn't stop seizing until the paramedics arrived. Thankfully, his van was unlocked. I zipped up his pants as I was tired of seeing his penis flop around."

"Thanks Officer James," I respond, stifling my laughter. I do a quick head to toe physical. Prying his eyelids open reveals both pupils equal and reactive to light. Heart and lungs sound normal. He had floppy extremities. Most people can fake soft, loosely hanging limbs. What they often are not able to do is disregard self-injury. What I mean by that is, most people can't turn off their self-protective instincts. I lifted up his right arm as high as it goes. I then positioned it over his nose. Next I drop his arm, so that if it has no muscle tone, it will strike his nose. Patients who are malingering will move their arm slightly to avoid smacking their noses or face area. When I drop his arm, the hand smacks hard into his nose. He doesn't move a muscle or wince in the least. Next, I grab an 18-gauge needle and stick it in the arch of his bare left foot. Nothing! No response whatsoever. I still have my doubts about this being a real seizure, but I have to assume the worst, even though my gut tells me this man was faking. Brain bleed is top of the unfavorable conditions that could cause a seizure. I mentioned this back when I had the lidocaine toxicity seizure patient. I order a CT head, blood work, and a urine drug screen. "Dave throw in a foley. No lido gel," I order. Even with numbing gel, most men react when a tube is pushed up their penis. Dave slides the catheter inside his urethra and he doesn't move a muscle. With not moving with the foley placement, that totals three negatives on the malingering diagnosis possibility. If this guy is faking, he might be as good an actor as Tom Hanks in his prime, that being Hank's entire career. "Send him to CT and get a lumbar puncture kit ready. When he returns, I'll do the LP." Jane the CT tech wheels him away with Dave accompanying.

I walk back to my desk and hear a chart hit the rack. Picking up the clipboard for Room 9, I read: CC: anal growths 18 y.o. female

What a lovely complaint, yeah not really. I look around for Sharon, Judy, or Melody. If I have neglected to inform you before, I will now. Physicians take a chaperone when examining patients of the opposite sex. That chaperone isn't always a nurse, but is the same sex as the patient. We do this 100% of the time for complaints involving the genitalia or female breasts. I also made a habit of doing it for suspected male homosexual patients. Of course these days with better awareness of LGBTQ rights, I attempt to never be alone when examining any sensitive areas. It provides the patient a confidant and limits any liability issues with what a patient might complain having occurred behind closed doors. To the non-medical person this might seem overly cautious. Let me share an unfortunate encounter one of my ED partners experienced.

This incident occurred during a very busy shift. One of our younger ED physicians was trying to be efficient and helpful when the waiting room started to overflow. There were no more ED beds available, so he started seeing and treating patients in the waiting room. This can be a common occurrence during busy hours or entire holiday weekends in any ER. Anyway, the young doctor decided to use the bereavement room to examine patients. This is the room where we talk to families when patients die or are likely to die. It offers loved ones some form of privacy to grieve without being in the middle of a loud chaotic ED. He wanted to provide some privacy to examine an abdominal pain patient and not expose her to fellow waiting room area people. The patient happened to be a middle-aged woman, and he was a young good looking male doctor. Looks and age shouldn't matter but are included for your edification. He made one mistake. He examined her abdomen without a chaperone. I have done this hundreds of times. However, this turned out to be a mistake because it was in a room outside of the ED and the patient was overly sensitive, vindictive, or evil. Exact details vary, but when he palpated her belly, he touched her breast. At least that is what the patient brought up in her complaint to the hospital. He denied touching her breast, but the end result was his banishment from working at that hospital. Of note is the fact that the majority of ED physicians are not employed by the hospital in which they work. How can that be, you may ask. Well emergency medicine groups are contracted to staff most hospital EDs across the country. Also, a high percentage of ED physicians work as independent contractors. In fact, since I finished residency, I have worked at a total of eight hospitals in four different states. (Counting residency, 16 hospitals in six states. If you include my four years being a medical student, you would have to double both numbers. I took advantage of the travel option during school). Not one of those hospitals has ever paid me a cent. I am employed by the emergency medicine group that staffs those EDs. Those ED groups are at the mercy of a hospital's decision. The ED group doesn't want to lose a contract and the hospital has no loyalty to a physician who they do not directly employ. In my colleagues' situation, the patient stipulated all she wanted was the doctor not to work at the ED anymore and she wouldn't pursue legal action. Our group didn't want to get attorneys involved, and we had another hospital that the wronged physician could switch to full time. He played ball and switched hospitals. I'm not saying he made a bad decision, but he didn't put up a fight. Personally, I would have hired my own attorney, burned some bridges, and stood my ground. The important point is, if he had a chaperone, then it would not have been her word against his.

I spot Melody and attempt to get her attention. Before I am able, Officer James gets mine. "Doc, I'm heading out now. Have a good night."

I responded, "Thanks officer. Do we need to call and update you on findings for our dude?"

She waves her hand at me. "No need. I hope he is ok. Even if he is faking, I wasn't going to ticket him. I was going to tell him to button up his pants and hit the road. I only wanted the prom kids to have a fun night free of weirdos." Officer James walks away.

Resuming my prior plan to get Melody's attention, I turn and almost bump into her protruding belly. "Sorry Melody, I need an escort for Room 9. Lead the way if you please." Even late in a busy shift, I try to picture the concerns of my patient. I'm pretty sure a teenage girl with an anal issue would rather see a pregnant woman come through the doors before a male doctor.

We arrive outside Room 9 and I defer to Melody. She knocks, and we hear, "Come in." Melody turns the knob and walks in. I let her take a few strides before I follow. A nicely dressed middle-aged woman is standing at the bedside. A younger version of her is sitting on the exam bed wearing a pink sweatshirt and matching pink sweatpants. The resemblance is remarkable. Without a doubt I know that the person standing at the bedside is the patient's mom.

"Hi guys, I'm Dr. Adams and this is Nurse Melody. Do you want to tell me why you are here or just show me?" Of course, having minimal patience, I always want to see the problem right away. Honestly, I couldn't care less about hearing most of the details. Often those details are only needed if the diagnosis isn't obvious.

In a shaky voice, the young woman says, "Mom you can tell him while I show him."

Very efficient. I try not to judge, but I like this patient. I put on some exam gloves as Melody assists the young girl, turning her to lay prone, and grabs a sheet to cover the patient's lower half. Before the mom starts talking I ask, "Is she sexually active?"

The mother answers, "Not really, but let me explain. My Shelly came home from prom tonight crying. She initially didn't want to talk about it, but then she gave me a full confession." I was listening as Melody pulled the sweat pant bottoms down exposing the girl's buttocks. I nodded to Melody to spread the patient's butt cheeks. The mother continued. "Shelly's anal area has been itchy lately, but tonight it started to bleed a little. I think she has..."

"Anal warts," I interrupt. I was looking down at a bunch of small protrusions near her anal opening. It is pretty surprising to see them on such a young woman. Equally shocking was her bleached anus. Her anus was an unnatural pale white, which made the six or seven anal warts more noticeable. I'm now positive Shelly has been sexually active.

"I told you, Mom," Shelly starts crying. I need to reassure them and hurry to check the results of the CT head of seizing masturbation man.

I begin my explanation and education. "Anal warts or condyloma are caused by HPV, the human papillomavirus. It is the most common sexually transmitted disease. She has been sexually active."

The young girl pulls her sweat pants up, turns over, and sits up. She then says, "I don't do vaginal. So, in God's eyes I'm still a virgin."

What the hell did she just say? I look at Melody, who looks equally confused. I don't know what to say to her response. I had never heard of such a thing. I decide that she can think whatever she wants, but I need to inform her of treatment options and check on my other patient. "I will write a cream medicine that you apply to the warts. If they get larger or continue to bother you, they can be surgically removed. Often they go away on their own, but can take up to a year or more. Even though you already have HPV, you could still get the new HPV vaccination that came out not that long ago. It can still provide protection from other strains you don't yet have."

I was going to leave it at that, but young Shelly speaks up. "Would the vaccine have protected me from getting these warts?" I could tell Shelly's mom is not happy about her daughter's inquiry. I would have tread more lightly, but my patience from this emotionally exhausting shift was fleeting.

"It's 90% effective against anal warts and more importantly up to 90% preventative for cervical cancer. Incredibly, it is a vaccine that saves people from contracting cancer," I inform her.

"Mom why didn't I get the vaccine?" Shelly asks.

"Well, I thought you would wait until marriage to have sex and not use God's loophole. God created your body to fight disease, and heal itself, you don't need any vaccinations. As simple as that," her mom harrumphs.

I doubted anything I was about to say would sway Shelly's mother, but Shelly might benefit from a little assistance. As a physician I have been trained in science and critical thinking. I also believe in God and feel strongly that these beliefs are not mutually exclusive. Years before the Covid pandemic the anti-science Christians were a source of irritation. I often give patients medical information and let common sense determine their choices. When patients seem to be lacking common sense, I provide insight based on the most updated medical science. Back then, I developed a few phrases, informing patients of the supporting facts. They could discard my words or consider my ideas later when they returned home. In this instance, I felt that Shelly might benefit from one of those concepts that dealt with fear of vaccinations. In her case I used an opinionated spin. After all, I didn't knock on their doors and force my beliefs on them. They came to my place of work and wanted my medical expertise. So, I said, "Well my God created all humans and amongst some of them he bestowed very high levels of intelligence. Some of those brilliant humans developed vaccinations to protect his precious creatures from suffering and death. My personal belief is God put knowledge and skills in their heads to help his flock and to deny their gifts would be an affront to God. That's my opinion, you are entitled to your own." Shelly's mom stood open-mouthed to my comments. On the other hand, Shelly's eyebrows were raised in a more contemplative expression.

Usually my personal opinions are highly based on medical science as well as years of experience. They deal with many issues other than vaccinations; diet and exercise, personal hygiene, sleep habits, substance abuse including alcohol use are only some of the topics my patient recommendations include. With an apparent lack of common sense at an all time high, you might think I would be using my medical based suggestions more often than ever. Sadly, the opposite is the case.

As a physician, providing medical education is a large part of my job description. I hesitate to bring it up but the recent Covid pandemic has negatively affected the way physicians provide that education. Part of the difficulty stems from politicians regardless of party, fighting to see who can have the tightest grip using medical fear as choke holds. Political ideology should not play a role in how physicians practice medicine. Unfortunately its effects are apparent. My partners have shown less patience and even less compassion since we moved through these medically challenging past few years. I am also guilty. Let me provide a simple example to demonstrate my point. During the first twenty years of my medical career, I made it a habit to tell patients to quit if they smoked. I might not ask every patient I saw if they smoked, but if I learned that they did smoke, I would give them a simple recommendation to stop. It usually came out in one of three ways: I would ask patients about their medical history and they would tell me, "Doc, I have diabetes" or "I have high blood pressure," or "No medical problems," etc. I would get to asking their social history which includes being married or single, if they drank alcohol and how much per week, and if they smoked and how many packs a day. Usually, we would double the drinking number as most patient's underestimate the amount of alcohol consumption, or just plain lie. The amount of packs per day a patient admits too is a little more accurate. What was important to me was not the amount, but if they did or didn't smoke. When a patient said yes to the question, "Do you smoke?" my response about 75% of the time was simply, "Quit." As simple as that, a one second response and then I moved on. If a family member were present with the patient and I could sense an unhappiness with the individual's smoking habit, I often would expand and say something like, "Best interest to you and your family if you stopped." Maybe a three to five second response. Lastly, if I sensed the patient was especially stubborn or in wretched health, I would say, "If you DON'T want to live a long and healthy life, continue." I would nonchalantly give my statement and then move right along with my next question. This may not be a nice way to motivate patients, but it's a more memorable rejoinder. The glaring fact of the matter is, the single most important health decision a smoker can make is to quit smoking. If I, as their physician—however fleeting my role in the ED was—didn't address the most important health decision regarding my patient, I would feel like I was doing an inadequate job.

Since we have come through the pandemic, I am ashamed to admit a fact. I now rarely tell my smoking patients to quit. Americans are now more defensive and argumentative than ever before. They don't come to me to be lectured or for my opinion on their social activities. They want me to fix the problem that brought them in and let them return home to live their life. I am in the business of fixing problems and putting out the metaphorical fires, not starting them. Thus, in order to limit conflict, I've changed the way I practice. My complacency is disconcerting. Worse than my behavior change, hell, I'm old and held off burn out for many years, is the many younger physicians that I witness show a similar growing apathy and that fact saddens me.

Melody and I walk back to my desk so I can write up a script for anal wart cream. I am waiting to see if Melody brings up any of the recent conversation or if I should. "Doc, what the hell is God's loophole?" Melody asks.

"Melody, today's the first time I have ever heard the term, but I think it's young girls having anal sex and not doing vaginal entry for religious reasons. I had friends growing up who always went after the preacher's daughters. Maybe that's why?" I laugh at that thought but inside feel a little dirty. I type up my anal wart patient's discharge and prescription. I pull up the results of my possible seizing beat off dude. Everything is normal. CT brain showed no acute findings, drug screen negative, blood work is pristine. I'm thinking that the chances the lumbar puncture shows anything is nil. I need to be thorough and other than him trying to get out of a ticket and a trip to jail, I have no other reason for his seizure. I walk back to Room 6 and see if Dave can report any change with the voyeur van man.

"Dave, anything to report?" I ask as I enter the room. The patient is lying supine with normal breathing and looks like he is resting comfortably.

"Nothing Doc, he hasn't budged. Jane from CT needed my help to slide him into the scanner. He's like a sack of potatoes." Before I was about to roll him onto his side, I thought I would take one last shot in the dark and mention that the officer left. So, in a loud voice I state, "Dave the police officer went home, so if our patient here makes a full recovery he would be free to go."

Dave and I are both silently praying as we look at the jerk off guy. Like a bolt of lightning, he sits up and says, "Did you say the cop is gone?" I look at Dave and smile. Our job is done. No LP for this wanker.

"Yes, the officer went home. She told me she only wanted to warn you and have you vacate the premises so the prom kids wouldn't be creeped out. That was it," I inform him.

He looks at me and Dave then responds with, "I'm sorry guys. I freaked because I didn't want to go to jail. I didn't mean to waste your time. I was really scared is all. I know I was doing something wrong. Man, I'm sorry."

He was so sincere that I believe him, but he could have been continuing his Oscar worthy acting skills on us. Either way, we had already wasted enough time on him, so I point to the exit and say, "There's the door, have a good night."

Dave was shaking his head as he says, "Let me deflate your foley catheter before you walk out. Pretty sure you don't want that as a souvenir."

When I finally did get around to my charts, what I wrote down as this patient's official diagnosis was pseudo-seizure secondary to incarceritis. In layman's terms it means a sham seizure brought on by threat of arrest or jail time. This occurs so often that the term "incarceritis" has been listed in the urban dictionary for some time.

I walk back to my desk as I look down at my watch. It was after 3:00 a.m. Less than three hours to go. No problem. No way could things get any more deranged. The night had thrown its most bizarre patients at me and I'm still fighting strong. Nothing else that comes my way could be more demented than what I've already experienced. Once again I was to be proven wrong.

Sharon brings me the next patient chart. "Doc, I'm going to go in with you when you see this patient." Why in all that is holy is Sharon so excited to see this particular patient at 3:20 a.m.? I grab Room 7's clipboard from her extended hand and look down.

CC: green dick and pissing razor blades 41 y.o. male

"You gotta be kidding me!" I moan. I have had patients complain of pissing razor blades before, but this was my first patient with a green penis complaint.

Sharon looks at me with a kooky grin and says, "Doc, I have never seen a green dick before." That makes two of us. The only difference is, I'm not nearly as psyched to see my first green cock as she is.

As Sharon and I walk toward Room 7, I think back to the most memorable time a patient told me he felt like he was pissing razor blades. It was during my residency years and I was working a shift at our small ER urgent clinic. The facility was located downtown in an undesirable area of the city. We opened at 8AM and closed at midnight. We fled every night before the clock struck 12. We did our best Cinderella impression of trying to avoid danger in the same way she wanted to prevent her carriage from turning back into a pumpkin. We wanted to steer clear of the dangerous night life that arose at the bewitching hour. Basically, we were a glorified sixteen-hour STD clinic.

The humorous patient encounter occurred during a quiet shift. The largest man I have ever seen walking on his own two feet entered the clinic. I qualify this because I once experienced a non-ambulatory patient weighing over a thousand pounds. This walking individual was as healthy looking as humanly possible for someone over 500 pounds. He was a well-dressed, enormous black man at least 6 and a half feet tall. Impossible to believe, but he would have made the legendary Chicago Bears football player William 'Refrigerator' Perry look like a mini-fridge. He was quickly triaged by our lone nurse, giving his razor blade when peeing description. I cautiously introduced myself because to put it plainly, his massive stature scared the hell out of me. "Hello, I'm Dr. Adams and usually when you're urination feels razor sharp, it indicates a gonorrheal infection." He tipped his head down and his huge mouth turned into a frown. "Is this the first time?" I asked.

Surprisingly, he answered, "No Doc, it's not. Six months ago, I had the same thing." What surprised me by his response was not that this problem was a recurrence, but that his voice was so high pitched and gentle. The giant continued, "I came here and you guys gave me a shot and some pills. I was better until yesterday when it started up again." As he tells me his story, a small shiver runs through my body. I forgot to explain that my attending physician also staffed the clinic with me. I use the term "staff" instead of "work" because they are usually in the back watching movies or doing fun activities while the doctor in training actually sees the patients. After an initial patient evaluation, I go to the back room and tell my attending the possible diagnosis and treatment plan, and he counsels me. My fear is that he will advise me to do a urethral swab on my colossal individual. Generally, what takes place when someone has a straightforward complaint and the diagnosis seems obvious is to provide treatment. We don't waste time and money doing tests. However, a reoccurrence or unclear diagnosis often warrants studies. In the case of infections, those studies are in the form of bacterial cultures. We can and do some viral and fungal testing, but by far bacterial testing is our focus. The body fluids we culture include urine, sputum, stool, blood, joint or synovial fluid, cerebral spinal fluid, or discharge from wounds or any human orifice. Depending on the laboratory and what is tested, the results can be reported in as early as an hour or as long as days. They report what organisms grow out—the specific bacterium if only one organism grew out or sometimes multiple bacteria. In addition, the lab reports what antibiotic showed sensitivity or can kill our bug or was resistant and won't harm that organism. So, when a patient calls two days later and says, "My symptoms haven't improved," we can look up the culture report and check if we prescribed the correct antibiotic. If the culture results show that the bacterium was resistant to our initial drug prescribed, we change it to one that is sensitive and should kill it. Bacteria develop resistance over time and this varies geographically. In the past, my mountain man was treated based on probable bug and antibiotic most likely to kill it. Chances are he has been reinfected, but after describing his case to my supervisor, my fears become reality. My attending physician told me to do the urethra swab. Current urine testing is nearly as accurate as the placing of a cotton swab an inch inside the tip of the penis and doing a quick twirl. Unfortunately, we didn't have the urine testing available back then. I still asked my attending, "Dr. Allen, did you see the size of this guy?"

With a straight face he responded, "The patient's size has nothing to do with the decision to do a urethra swab test." He's having fun at my expense. Hours later, the nurse would confirm my suspicion when she told me it had been over a year since Dr. Allen had last used a urethral swab.

I walked warily back into my patient's exam room. I calmly informed him that the quick test procedure gave the most precise culture possible. I then showed him the swab I was going to use. His falsetto response was, "DOC YOU GOING PUT THAT IN MY PEE PEE?" I had to bite my tongue. My fear of this massive human being coupled with his near glass shattering high pitched voice was so surreal it filled me with the urge to laugh uncontrollably. While I was suppressing my over emotional reflex, he consented to the testing, "Ok, if you gotta. But you gotta hold it as I can't look." I had to bite my tongue even harder, as I wasn't sure how he would respond if I laughed while he exposed his penis and placed it in my hands. He then pulled out his impressive appendage. "Doc, this is going hurt bad, right."

I didn't want to lie, but I also didn't want to die. I skirted the question, by telling him, "It will be quick." The test took two seconds. He shed a single tear while covering his mouth and eyes with his two enormous hands. I gave him a 1 gram intramuscular dose of Rocephin and oral antibiotics for home. We treat both Gonorrhea and Chlamydia at the same time. They can often occur simultaneously, and we don't want to wait one or two days to get results back before treating. The cultures would later confirm the Gonorrhea. It is the second most common notifiable communicable disease in the U.S., behind Chlamydia. This means health providers are required to report it to state or local health officials. In truth, the hospital lab or hospital liaison reports it, doctors don't. We only probe the painful prick and sometimes hold it too.

I knock and walk into Room 7 with Sharon a step behind me. Sitting on the exam bed completely naked with a sheet balled up over his crotch is my next patient. He didn't really need to take his shirt off, especially with Room 7 being the coldest room in the department. *I'm a bit worried by his exhibitionism.* His extensively black hairy chest and limbs do give the appearance that he can handle more cold than most naked individuals. His leathery face makes him look much older than his age. "I'm Dr. Adams and you met Nurse Sharon. You want to show me the problem?" He didn't answer, he just placed the balled sheet behind his back revealing a very small penis. The penis was mostly hidden by the massive amount of jet-black pubic hair. I actually had to take a few steps closer to see what the color of his penis was. Other than the small size, what made it difficult to see was its dark green tint was hidden by his pubic hair. When I neared, I realized it had a mixture of green colors—a darker army green combined with a slightly lighter grass green pigmentation. Remember earlier when I said I didn't need details, only to look at the problem? Well, this time I needed the details. I had no idea why this man had a green penis. All I knew was if it burned with urination—medical term is dysuria—then infection was likely. "When did it turn green?" I ask.

The usually chatty Sharon is speechless waiting for the patient's response. He is tight lipped as well, but quietly says, "Couple weeks now."

There is more to the story, but he isn't ready to divulge all the details. I continue, "Did anything happen a couple weeks ago that could help explain the color and why it burns when you urinate?"

He looks over at Sharon and I can sense he feels uncomfortable talking in her presence. I am surprised by this as he had no apprehension with exposing himself in her company.

"Would you prefer to talk with me alone?" He nods in reply. I wave Sharon away. As she walks out the door she gives me the, "You better tell me all the details later" look. Leaving the two of us alone, I say, "You can cover yourself back up and put your shirt on." He nonchalantly puts his shirt on first, then grabs the sheet and plops it on his crotch area. With Sharon gone, things will not get any more comfortable than they were. Now I can cut to the chase. "I am not here to judge you. I need to know what you think might have turned your penis green so I can treat it and make it better." He slowly lets out a sigh and sits back in the bed. The words had hit their mark and now I only need to wait. I pull up a chair and sat down. You already know I am very impatient, but some situations call for restraint. If I forcefully tried to reel him in like an amateur fisherman, this patient would fall off the hook.

Sitting on my stool in the cold exam room, I stare at this hairy fellow, both of us saying and doing nothing. This was the hardest thing I had done all shift. After what felt like twenty minutes but was probably two or three, he finally opens his mouth, "Doc, I've been having sex with Billy." He stops there and doesn't elaborate. I already figured sex or placing his penis inside something was the cause of his problem. The information he offered doesn't provide me with enough information to answer our dilemma.

I need more, so I push a little. "Who is Billy and how long has this been going on?" I study his response as I hope the hook was still secure but I know he could still detach and break free at any time.

His body relaxes completely and his lips turn down forming a frown. He had resigned to his fate. "About one month now, and um Billy…Billy is my brother's goat."

Holy shit balls! I nearly fell off the stool. A flood of quandaries hit me at once. Do I report this to the police? What bacteria are in a goat's anus? Does the goat hold still? Focus and hold off on any judgment. This was now the most difficult task of the entire shift. I really like animals. I love dogs and tolerate cats. Goats are pretty damn cool too. And this guy is a goat fucker. Argh! I take a breath and form my problem list in my head. Do I need to legally report this? I have no idea. I know bestiality is against the law, but I don't know if it is a felony or misdemeanor or even my responsibility to report. This wasn't covered in med school or residency. There are only a few things we have to report 100% of the time: any gunshot wound, any non-self-inflicted stabbing, and child or elder abuse of any type. That's my legal physician list—short and not sweet. There are other reportable situations, but they vary by state and institution. I was in a quandary on bestiality. Most other reportable events deal with common protection of people and not stepping over their freedoms. The key word here is "people." I decided not to call the police.

On to problem two, the infection. Once again, I am in a unique predicament. I have no idea what bugs were in a goat's anal area. His green color appearance I surmised came from the goats mostly grass diet. The fact that he has a burning sensation upon urination likely indicates an infection. I am thinking Billy probably wasn't a promiscuous goat, so a sexual transmitted disease (STD) is less likely. In all seriousness, I doubted the usual STDs, Gonorrhea or Chlamydia, are the culprit. An abdominal gut bacterium could be the source, but I am only attempting to make an educated guess. I end up doing urethral swabs and treating him with an IM dose of one antibiotic, and an IV dose of another, and starting him on two different oral doses of antibiotics for home. I will check the culture results in one or two days and modify my treatment plan accordingly.

For the third dilemma of how this perverted act transpired, I decide it would be better to not have an answer. I figure if he gave me a detailed description, I will have a visual image burned into my memory banks for the rest of my life. I already have more than enough awful visuals to last a lifetime.

No matter how many years a health professional works in the ED, they haven't seen everything. Nobody has or ever will. Thank goodness! Most doctors and nurses will have a string of shifts without seeing anything totally new or different. After a while, an ER worker might start wishing for that unique or strange presentation. I am at the point in my career where I no longer want the completely unheard of or unbelievable case. I know that regardless of my feelings, the never-seen-before patient will eventually show up. They always do!

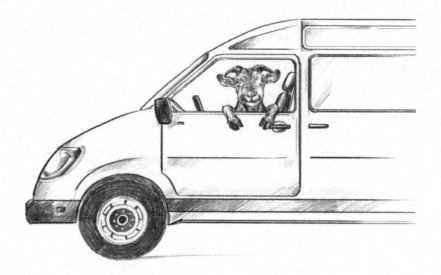

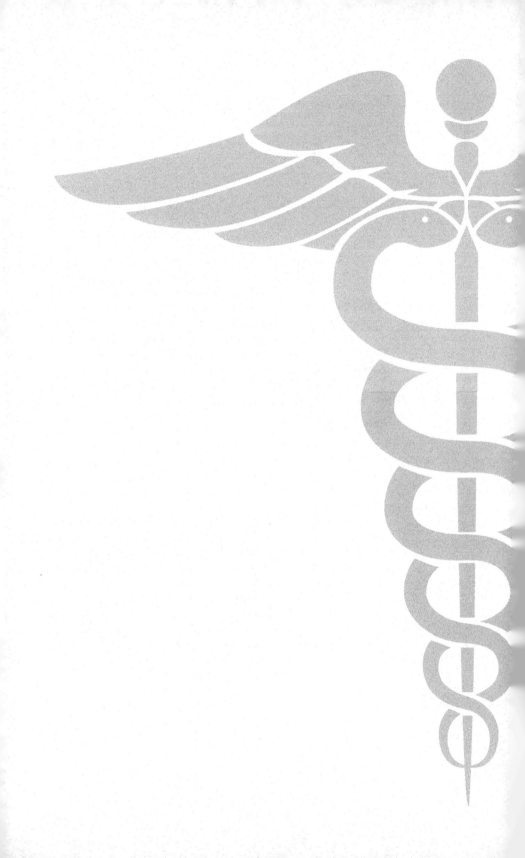

CHAPTER 9

What the F*** is stuck? 3:42 a.m.

Dave yells from the triage area, "Doc, I need you in triage!" I was sitting at my desk giving Sharon the minimal details I had on our recent goat fornicator. I had kept Sharon in the dark until she had medicated him. Now that he was waiting for meds to infuse before discharge, I was spilling the beans. She is professional, but her love of animals would have made her vengeful. Usually, my nurses protect me from getting too emotional. This time I was the protector. "Doc, come to triage, I need help," Dave cries out again.

Man, I'm tired. I have to stand up and find out what Dave wants. "I'm coming Davey," I answer back.

Experienced nurses know when to shout for the doctor. The terrible vitals, apneic, and pulseless patients I need to be informed immediately. However, the psychotic, drug fueled, or aggressive patient is trickier. Outside the ER, when someone gets ready to fight, the gloves come off. When I get called to race to an exam room, ready to fight, the gloves come on! I will order knock out medication, four-point leather restraints, security, and possibly police. I'm decent at talking some people down, but many times it is pointless or even dangerous to delay the inevitable, which is to take them down and control them as fast and safely as possible. Remember earlier when I alluded to the 2 x 4 piece of lumber? I usually decide which way to go in about one or two seconds.

I rapidly make my way into triage. Dave is trying to pull an older woman away from the wall. She is attempting to bang her head against a cement pillar. "Doc, she told me bugs are trying to chew into her brain." Dave's hands were full, but he still should have called a Code Strong. Hospitals have special overhead signals to indicate certain emergent needs. A well- known example is a Code Adam for a missing child or infant. That is universal, even outside of the hospital. The hospital uses Code Pink for stolen or lost infants. Dave could have called either a Code Strong, which informs staff to come to help for a possibly a cognitively challenged patient, or a lift assist is needed. Or, he could have called a Code Grey, for an abundance of man power to overwhelm and physically subdue a combative patient.

"KYLE AND JASON TO TRIAGE!" I yell. I grab the woman's left arm so Dave can focus exclusively on her right arm. We successfully move her away from the wall.

"Aaahhh! They're eating into my brain. Aaahhh!" the woman screams as we escort her to Exam Room 1. Patients come in every week with the complaints of bugs crawling on or out of their skin. This is termed, "formication." It manifests commonly in opiate and alcohol withdrawal, or while taking stimulants, usually methamphetamines. Occasionally, I have patients describe bugs crawling into their skin but never have they said eating into their brain. This lady looks to be in her seventies. She is wearing a nice nightgown and has spotless hygiene as far as I can tell. Something is not adding up here.

"Dave, did someone bring her or is she alone?" We place her onto an exam bed. The head of the bed is angled up, so she doesn't have to lay flat.

"Doc, she walked into the waiting room moaning. I pulled her straight into triage. She didn't have any ID and no one was with her," Dave confesses.

Jason and Kyle arrive to assist. I let the muscular Kyle take my place securing the mentally unstable woman. I position myself so my face is directly in front of hers. "Ma'am, are you alone?" She doesn't answer me. "Jason, run out to the waiting room and find out if anybody brought a hysterical older woman," I order.

As Jason starts his sprint toward the waiting room, I spot Judy escorting an older gentleman toward us. He is dressed in an equally high- quality nightgown that matches my psychotic acting senior citizen. "Doc, this is her husband. She has something stuck in her ear," Judy informs me. Oh man, now things make a lot more sense.

"Dave, grab 2 mg of Ativan. Kyle, can you hold her head absolutely still? I'm gonna take a quick look." I grab the otoscope and screw on a disposable plastic speculum tip. Not only are otoscopes shaped to look in ear canals, but they also provide up to forty times magnification. She seems to be wincing and scratching more at her left ear, so that becomes my first choice to inspect. While Kyle is using his huge forearms to lock her head in place, I place the otoscope tip in her left ear canal. I look in and something looks right back at me. I have to fight the impulse to jump backwards. It was some kind of insect.

"Oh God, it stopped. My brain is safe," the woman starts crying in relief. I pull out the otoscope to inform Judy or Dave to get me a special forceps, alligator type. As soon as I withdrew my otoscope, "Aaahhh! it's going for my brain again!" The insect must have turned back around to resume tunneling into her tympanic membrane, or eardrum.

"Doc, got the alligator forceps," Judy announces. The tip of the forceps is shaped like an alligator's mouth, thus its name. They are small enough to be placed in tight spaces while allowing the operator to open, advance, close, then retract. Hopefully after retracting, the foreign body is now in the alligator's mouth. Often it is not that simple, but I'm usually successful. Judy opens the bag containing the sterilized unique forceps. I grab the instrument and am hoping the Ativan effects will make my job easier. My bug inducing psychotic lady is still flopping around in the bed more than before. Dave had given her the Ativan sublingual, which means under her tongue. The oral mucosal absorption is quicker than the stomach and I wanted the fastest medication reaction without giving her any more trauma like an injection would. It had yet to achieve anything.

"Kyle, hold her head tight. Everybody else restrain her as gently as possible. Let's get this done on the first attempt," I instruct. Taking the otoscope, I slide the plastic magnified area slightly so I can introduce my forceps right into the otoscope. With the otoscope in my left hand and forceps in my right, I advance them into her ear canal simultaneously. This allows me to continue to see the magnified object while I grab it. The bug was snug up tight to her eardrum, wiggling. I open the forceps and push slightly forward.

"AAAHHH! IT HURTS!" my patient yells as I press on the bug that was already pressing on her sensitive eardrum. I quickly, but not too quickly, close the alligator mouth onto the little bastard. I retract the otoscope and the entire insect is in the jaws of my alligator's choppers.

"Yes!" I say. One attempt and I had grabbed what looked like a cockroach-type insect, fully intact, wings and all. The damn thing was still alive and twitching in what looked like its death throes.

"Oh God. It's over, right?" my exhausted patient asks while looking up, recognizing her husband's presence for the first time. She embraces her husband, wrapping her arms around his rotund belly. "Oh Papa, it's passed. It really felt like it was trying to burrow into my brain. I felt like I was going crazy," the relieved elderly patient admits.

I quickly type up her discharge and have the nurse dispense an antibiotic ear drop for home. There was no current infection, but the little bugger had caused some trauma to her canal and ear drum. A prophylactic medicine would also provide her an added psychological reassurance. I hand the nurse the paperwork when Sharon announces, "We have another one!"

Another patient after 4AM, why would they stop now. Sharon wasn't alluding to just another patient, but to a specific type of another one. "Doc, I'll put her in Room 2. She also has a bug in her ear," Sharon informs me. What are the odds? Well, these problems occur when people lay their head down to sleep, so odds increase on the night shift. I walk into Room 2 and see another elderly patient in a nightgown.

"Hi, I'm Dr. Adams. What are you feeling in your ear?"

She calmly responds with a pleasant smile, "Hi Doc. I'm pretty sure a bug either crawled or flew into my left ear, but I think it's dead now. It stopped moving after I poured water and jammed a Q-tip in a bunch of times."

I am pleasantly surprised at her matter-of-fact response. No need to call all hands to assist this patient. "Let me take a look before I get my special grabber tool," I respond. She did indeed have a similar looking insect, but more squished and wet appearing. It took me five or six attempts to remove everything as the damn thing broke off in parts. Eventually, I got all of it and discharged her with the same antibiotic. The only difference was I had caused most of the trauma to the skin of her ear canal, versus my earlier patient where I only needed one attempt.

I typed up the second FB ear removal patient for discharge and stood up with a plan to visit the restroom. I really needed to empty my bladder when Judy interrupted my plans with another chart.

Clipboard room 8: CC: can't urinate 13 y.o. female

"Doc, she looks really uncomfortable. Something isn't right with this poor girl," Judy confides.

Now if I make a quick trip to the bathroom, I'm going to feel guilty. So much for plans. I'll check on the teenage girl, then take care of my pressure problem. "Judy, lead the way to 8." I start thinking about the thirteen-year-old's complaint. Inability to urinate is a very common occurrence in the ED, especially on the night shift. This usually happens when older men develop Benign Prostatic Hyperplasia (BPH), a large prostate. Simple aging results in the prostate enlarging so much that pressure constricts the urethra and a dam is created. Infection or medication can also contribute, but all men over eighty will develop an enlarged prostate with over half resulting in urinary retention difficulties. Women can experience urine retention, but to a much lesser frequency. In younger people it is very rare and the causes vary. I did know a thirteen-year-old girl with a terrible history of kidney stones. She would have moderate difficulty urinating every time she was trying to pass stones. Every male member of her family had a history of kidney stones. This genetic inheritance caused her to visit the ER every six months, where she would get pain med assistance to pass the larger stones. Every time I treated her, I brought up the fact that when she gets older and starts a family, she won't be asking for an epidural during labor.

I let Judy lead the way into the room. The teenager is leaning up against the exam bed as she looks too uncomfortable to sit down. A woman who I presume is her mom, is sitting in one of the chairs next to her. I give the mother a smile, then look toward the patient. "Hello, I'm Dr. Adams. How long have you been having problems urinating?"

The young woman looks down at her mom for help with answering my question. "Honey, you can tell the doctor. He is here to help," the mother reassures.

"I've been having problems for a couple of days, but today I only got dribbles out, and my back started hurting."

Before I walked in, my probable diagnosis list had already begun. Now with back pain as an added symptom, my list is growing. "Judy, can you do a bladder scan and we can see how much our patient is retaining," I instruct. Turning to the patient, I ask her, "Can I check your belly and back?" She nods and reluctantly slides into the bed. I lower the head portion so she is completely flat. Her face grimaces. "Lift your knees up, this will take some pressure off your back," I explain as I place a pillow under her now bent knees. She looks younger than her thirteen years. Her build is slightly on the chubby size, but her baby looks give her the appearance that she has yet to grow into her body. I put my hands on her belly without lifting her sweatshirt. I figure better to take it slow, and a simple test I had already planned to have Judy perform would expose her abdomen soon enough. As I gently lay my hands over her belly, I am surprised at how distended she actually is. Her expanded portion is her lower abdomen, the supra pubic and down to the pelvic area. This is similar to what I palpate when older gentlemen's prostate causes severe urinary retention. Next I put my hand under her low back and her normal lordotic curve is gone. I have to push hard into the firm mattress to get under her back to reach her spine. This is something common in obese patients. She isn't that tender, but doesn't like the pressure that I added to her spine. Something else might be pushing on her spine as a full bladder alone usually would not do this. Judy wheels in the bladder scanner, which is basically a one function ultrasound that measures volume of urine in bladders. Judy lifts up the girl's sweatshirt showing a bulging belly mirroring a term pregnancy appearance. Judy then places the probe over the young woman's protruding bladder area. The girl winces with minimal pressure but doesn't cry out or move. This is hurting her more than she is admitting.

"Wow!" Judy and I both say as we look down at the volume read out of 900 cc of urine. At 1000 cc, a full liter, I've witnessed grown men sobbing, on more than one occasion. I look at the mom. "We need to put a catheter in and drain her bladder." Then it hit me, I haven't asked when or if she had started menstruating. Young girls are menstruating earlier every decade, with the most common age to start one's period around twelve years old. Girls as young as eight can start menstruation and on rare occurrences begin after age sixteen. Interestingly, age sixteen was the most common age to start menses a century ago. "How long ago did she start having periods?" I ask.

I look at mom and the young girl. The girl looked at me like I was speaking a foreign language. She has no idea what a period was. I look back over to her mom. "Um, she hasn't had any bleeding yet." Slightly unusual, but shouldn't affect the ability to urinate or not. Her lack of knowledge on menses at age thirteen was more atypical.

"I'm going to order an ultrasound of her pelvis and we'll send a urine sample after a foley catheter is placed," I inform everyone. I quickly stepped out of the room to give the patient a little privacy while Judy finishes setting up the foley catheter placement kit. I hand Cindy my few simple orders and head toward the restroom.

"Doc, please come back in here," Judy cries out. Damn it, my bladder feels like I have a liter to empty. The poor girl is half my size and probably retaining twice the urine I'm holding, suck it up for five more minutes.

I walk back into 8 and ask Judy, "What is it?" The young woman was in a frog leg position with a sheet covering her pelvis. The foley catheter bag was hanging on the bed rail half-filled and still draining. Great. I ask the young girl, "Now that the urine is draining, do you feel better?"

"Yes, my belly feels a ton better, but my back pain is still there," she answers. I look at a concerned Judy who is pointing at the patient's covered vaginal area. "Judy, what do you need to show me?" I could tell she wasn't sure how tactful she needed to be with whatever it was she wanted to reveal. Remember I'm not good at waiting. Deciding Judy isn't going to divulge her findings, I need to look for myself. I quickly put on a pair of gloves. "I'm going to have a look at where the foley is draining," I inform the patient and mother. Seeing the urine draining I knew that the urethra was probably fine, but Judy's nervous pointing had me concerned for something else.

I lift up the sheet and visually examine her vaginal opening. What I was looking for wasn't there. She had an imperforate hymen. Her entire vaginal opening was covered by mucosal tissue, the hymen. I now had the answer to her problem. The ultrasound would confirm, but my suspicion is that she had begun menstruating but the blood had no opening to exit. How many periods she may have already had, I didn't know. I did know that she would need my gynecologist, Big John, to do a surgical opening called a hymenotomy, also called a hymenectomy. My unlucky girl's diagnosis was something called hematocolpos. Roughly 1 in 1000 girls will be born with an imperforate hymen. Often this is discovered earlier and the surgical procedure is performed before they reach puberty. My young patient was a bit on the naive side and her mother's probably hands-off approach didn't help matters. I begin informing both of them, "Well, I know what is causing her urine retention. She has probably started her menses but the blood has no way to drain. The hymen is completely covering her vagina. We'll still get the ultrasound, but I need to have our gynecologist on call come and see her." I would let Big John explain the need for the surgical opening procedure and what that entails. They both have plenty of new information to digest in the mean time..

I walk out and ask Cindy to call Big John in about three minutes. That should give me enough time to empty my bladder unless something has overgrown my urethra from my delaying to void. I take care of my much-needed business and have a very gratifying walk back to my desk. I spot my chocolate chip cookies in the corner and realize how hungry I am. My bladder pain must have been overriding my hunger pains. I grab the cookies and sit down.

I take a big bite of one of the cookies and Cindy tells me, "Doc, Big John on Line 1."

Chewing rapidly, I pick up the phone, hoping I don't sound to gar-bled, and start talking, "John hope you got a nap after the torsion case. I have a thirteen-year-old with an imperforate hymen who couldn't pee. The foley cath drained almost 1 Liter. I'll have a nurse put in an IV to give sedation so you can make an opening and drain the blood." I paused to see if he was awake enough to comprehend all the garbled information I threw at him.

"Got it. Had a delivery after that girl's torsion surgery, so I was nap-ping in the call room. Be down in five," Big John concludes. Great, he is in house and will be able to provide the definitive treatment that my patient needs. I inform Judy to place an IV, and some Versed medication to be ready at bedside along with a consent form for the procedure.

I sit back and eat the other two cookies in a tranquility that lasts all of one minute. "Doc, Melody is bringing back a seventeen-year-old belly pain to Room 4. She is vomiting," Jason informs me. "Hey Doc, it's after 4, so Kyle and I are going to make sure the rig is prepped and clean for the next shift," Jason states. I wave to him as he and Kyle walk out the front doors of the ED. Basically, he was asking if it was ok if they take an hour or two nap until 6AM or possibly to 7AM when their shift ends. Typically, from 5 AM to 6 AM, the ER is pretty quiet. I am done at 6AM, so I am praying no more ambulance calls occur during my last two hours. I have my hands full dealing with the walk-in patients. Standing up and heading to Room 4, I think, if this new and hopefully last patient of the night is straight forward, I may start my charts before the end of my shift.

I walk into Room 4 and witness Melody starting an IV on a retching patient. The smell of vomit hits me like a wave crashing into shore. The source of the smell is a young woman wearing a very baggy purple sweat-shirt, and matching sweatpants. An older woman on the opposite side of Melody, is holding a half-filled vomit bag to the patient's mouth. I'm super impressed by Melody's ability to withstand the stench while being eight months pregnant and having hyper olfactory senses. "Hi, I'm Dr. Adams. Once Melody gets that IV in, we'll get you some nausea meds and start some fluids. That should help. When did the vomiting start and can you describe your belly pain?"

She wasn't in any shape to answer, but I was hoping the older woman, who I guessed was her mother, would. I look at the vomit bag holder and she starts talking. "I'm Jenny's mom and she started vomiting on the car ride here. Her pain started a couple hours ago and comes in waves." Now I have some information, but really I need to get the retching under control so I can examine her and get the description from her own vomit-covered mouth.

Pain in waves is often termed colicky. It is often sharp and can come on abruptly in spasm-like waves that can stop intermittently. There are three main types of problems that present to the ER with colicky pain. Very common are the biliary or gallbladder issues. A gallstone or even gallbladder infection causes irregular painful attacks. Equally common is renal issues. Kidney stones top the renal list with painful crescendos and waning dull pain descents. Lastly, intestinal issues from constipation to more severe complete bowel obstructions can have a spasmodic painful pattern. Most other abdominal problems, that are serious anyway, rarely wax and wane from hurting then stopping only to resume again. Thus, a patient's description and timing of pain help me focus on a possible diagnosis even before I lay my hands on them.

"Melody, give her 4 mg Zofran and 1 liter NS bolus. Jenny, when you are able, I need to check your belly and we need a urine sample. How long ago was your last period?"

Before Jenny answered me, she wiped the vomit from her mouth with the sleeve of the sweatshirt. "About one month ago, I guess. My bleeding was a little light." She said that her menses was less than normal. Meaning, she could have a very early pregnancy. That pregnancy might have implanted outside the uterus, now causing considerable pain. Ectopic pregnancy is always a possibility we ER Docs consider in any female abdominal pain patient, from ages eight to eighty. Well, around fifty years old, anyway. The main reason is that it can prove deadly. It usually isn't colicky in nature, but a quick urine or blood test is all I need to check it off the list.

"I'll be back in five minutes so you can clean up and to give time for the medication to work," I inform as I walk out of the nausea-inducing room. In the past, I have pushed on vomiting patient's abdomens with varied success at localizing their pain, but achieving to enhance their spewing.

I walk back to my desk and pick up a chart to dictate. "Doc, don't start dictating. Dave wheeled a man back to Room 3 and I kinda overheard his complaint," Cindy whispers over my shoulder. Telling me what to do is very unlike Cindy. She is usually great at staying in her lane. This doesn't bode well in the least.

Putting the chart back on the stack, I bite and ask, "So what is the new patient's problem?"

Cindy starts laughing, "You remember the stuck coke bottle we had a few months ago?"

I actually slap my forehead and answer, "No! I mean of course I recall. Well, I guess the night wouldn't be complete without a foreign body in the backdoor." Back in March, a middle-aged man had come in because the coke bottle he was using to stimulate himself had gotten lodged in his anal cavity. Autoeroticism is the most common reason for anal foreign body presentation to the ED. The key to removal is pretty much to follow what approach allowed entry. Usually, RELAXATION and DILATION to put it in, followed by RELAXATION and DILATION to pull it out. In the ED, the relaxation medications I have at my disposal is vast. The tools to assist dilation are equally impressive. After I sedated that prior individual, the surgeon dilated the anal opening. Once adequately dilated, or so we thought, we both worked the forceps to attempt removal. What had transpired was the open bottle was inserted with the top first, creating a suction that would not budge. We needed to drill a hole in the glass bottom to open the vacuum, thus nullifying the suction. We actually got a drill from maintenance and did this in the ED. Usually the OR is more appropriate. The friction from the drill did make the glass bottle heat, so we had a nurse spraying cool water into the gentleman's anal opening. The bidet nurse had a ringside seat to the show. Once the hole was drilled, the forceps removal of the bottle was smooth sailing.

Cindy interrupts my stroll down memory lane. "This one isn't a bottle. He stuck an avocado up his butt!"

I am speechless. Once I regain my composure, I ask Cindy a question I already knew the answer to. "Do we have GI (Gastrointestinal) on call at all this weekend?"

She looks at me and shakes her head. "Ok, give me a few minutes to attempt an avocado delivery. If I'm unsuccessful I'll have you call the surgeon in," I tell Cindy. I usually like treating foreign body removals, but as you can guess these types are not my favorite. I walk into Room 3 and see Dave starting an IV. A man about my age in a retro t-shirt and jean shorts is trying to lie perfectly still. His eyes are closed and his entire body is tensed up. "Hello, I'm Dr. Adams. Can you roll onto your belly so I can have a quick peek."

The patient opens his eyes a smidge. "I don't want to move, Doc. When I do, the spasms that shoot from my ass are extremely painful." I think I understand, but really have no idea at all what he is talking about. I always thought of myself as a guy who would try anything once. I'm pretty sure I don't want that description applying to me anymore.

"OK. Dave here will give you some IV Valium which is a great muscle relaxer. Then I'll take a look, ok?" I offer and ask him at the same time.

"That sounds good, Doc. Can you not tell everybody here what is wrong with me? I'm kinda embarrassed." This dude is embarrassed now?

After I call the surgeon to assist then he'll be truly mortified. I'm sure my surgeon will bring his entire entourage to serve him this time. He came alone earlier, but basically after 4 AM it is a new day as far as surgeons are concerned. I could attempt to do the entire procedure all by myself, but I am exhausted and not in the mood to do all the dilating. Also, if I mess it up and he needs to go to the operating room, the surgeon will be pissed if I made a mess of things. I love to make guacamole, but not while I'm on shift.

After Dave gave the Valium, the patient rolled onto his belly. I glove up and have Dave assist me by spreading the cheeks as far as we could. My initial digital exam comes up empty for any FB. Also, I was hoping to take a quick peek looking for any green color. I assume it wasn't ripe as many avocados can turn more black than a dark green when ripe. "Um, it isn't ripe yet I hope?" I gently poise the question.

He responds, "No, but now that it is in a dark place, it will ripen faster." Well at least he hadn't lost his sense of humor. A knock on the door refocuses me to the fact I'm looking for any green color up this dark shaft.

"Doc, it's Melody. The vomiting has stopped and her pain is nearly gone."

"Great, thanks," I respond. Then I realize Dave and I need another hand. "Melody, come in quick and close the door behind you." She takes one step into the room and stops. She was busy with her patient, and had no idea what we were currently doing in here. "We need you to aim the overhead light better, then glove up and help pull back his butt cheeks so I can again try to palpate something," I causally inform her. After a moment of hesitation, Melody aims the light, positions herself near Dave, and places her hands on the patient's bum cheeks.

Quietly, Melody mutters, "Um, what are we searching for?" With the extra hands opening the entrance wider, I reattempt a digital exam and am finally able to palpate the foreign body. "I can barely touch the avocado. I need to call the surgeon in, but hopefully he can get it out down here and not have to go up to the OR," I announce to everyone.

Melody and I throw our gloves away as I tell her to lead the short few steps back to 4. Melody begins informing me, "Big John is with Judy and wants you to order the sedation medicine so he can cut some girl's hymen. What is that about?" I give Melody a brief description and tell her I'll check on Judy and Big John and come straight back to our now vomit-free patient.

I dart over to Room 8 and give Judy the Versed order, tell her to call respiratory, and say "Hi" to Big John. "When everything is set let me know and I'll jump back in for the pushing of the sedation medicine," I tell them. I don't plan to stay for the entire procedure, as I have no idea how long it will take to open that unfortunate girl's vaginal covering. I swing by Cindy's desk and tell her to call the surgeon for me. "If I'm in a room, tell him it's a stuck anal foreign body. Only tell him what the foreign body is if he asks. He likes surprises," I laugh as I sprint back to Room 4.

I knock on Room 4's door and hear Melody say, "Come in." The young woman lying on the bed looks more comfortable and there is only a faint vomit smell lingering in the air.

"I need to check your belly. Is the pain gone?" I ask.

"Doc, I still feel bloated, but no intense pain anymore."

I look at Melody. "Have we got a urine sample yet?"

She answers, "Not yet, but I sent blood to the lab."

I'll have to add a serum pregnancy test as she may take a long time before providing urine. In the meantime, I need to examine her abdomen. I step to the exam bed and pull up her sweatshirt. Her belly is very distended and it immediately reminds me of the girl who Big John is about to operate on. What is going on? I push down on her right lower area, where I would expect her appendix to be located.

"Ouch!" she responds.

I push on the left side. "Ouch!" she repeats. I use the same pressure and at a totally different location and get the same reaction. More shocking is how firm her entire belly is.

A thought crosses my mind, so I have to ask, "Are you sure you aren't pregnant?"

The patient looks at her mom and her mom stares right back at her. "I am not pregnant," she says.

Her mother reiterates, "She's not pregnant. She hasn't even had sex yet."

The air seems to leave the room with that comment as the patient sits up in the bed. "Um Mom, Keith and I have been having sex, but he uses protection." I look at Melody and her bulging pregnant belly and look down at this girl's similar size and shaped abdominal area.

"Jenny! You better not let your dad find out. He'll kill Keith. I know he will." Jenny's mom confides.

"Oh God! Mom, you're right. Keith is out in the waiting room sitting next to dad. Please! Please don't say anything to Dad," Jenny begs.

"Jenny, I don't want your daddy to go to jail. I won't say nothin!" her mom promises.

While the conversation between mother and daughter continues, I ask Melody to grab a fetal heart rate (FHR) doppler. This enables me to listen for a baby's heart rate which should be much faster than the mothers. Fetal heart range is 120-160 beats per minute (BPM). The spot I usually start from to find the FHR is above the pubic bone. Trying to tune out mom and daughter's fearful conversation, I place the probe on the patient's pubic bone and move upward until I hear a heartbeat. I quickly locate a fast beat. I start counting and grab the patient's wrist to access her radial pulse. As I predicted, the radial pulse was much slower than the 170 on my fetal doppler.

"Mom, the doctor found my heartbeat in my belly." This young woman didn't strike me as an idiot, but her denial was incredible.

"Honey, that sounds pretty fast for your heart," her mom's comprehension became less clouded.

"Oh, God! It's starting to hurt again," the girl says while trying to sit up more in bed. I pulled off the doppler and step back at the perfect time. As soon as I am a step from the bed, a torrent of fluid gushed from between her legs. Her amniotic sac had ruptured. Well, if the fetal heart rate wouldn't convince them, hopefully this would erase any doubts. This woman's colicky pain is from the fact that she is in active labor.

"I am going to get the obstetrician, the baby doctor. You don't belong in my ER. We have a separate area of the hospital for this condition," I blurt. I ran out of the room to inform Big John. If I had a white flag to wave, my right arm would be raised high, shaking back and forth. I can handle blood, guts, death, dismemberment, rotting tissues, and every smell that goes along with them, but faced with the act of having to deliver a baby, I run for the hills. Truthfully, I want to run, but in actuality I shake in my shoes. I am not afraid to admit that a woman in labor is the last type of patient I want in my ED. It is not a completely irrational fear. Some of my dread stems from an early incident that left a scar. It occurred while I was finishing my last few medical school rotations—specifically, my required obstetrics and gynecology month. I had attempted to spend more time in the OR doing the gynecology surgeries, not because I loved the OR, but I was trying to avoid the obstetric or childbirth portion of my rotation. The doctor with whom I was working finally figured out why I was always eager to assist in the OR. So, he told me that during my last week, I would be assisting him with every patient who went into labor. His idea of me assisting meant that I did the delivery myself while he stood at bedside and watched.

The first laboring patient of that dreadful week was a young woman about nineteen or twenty years old. She wasn't married, but her devoted baby daddy was at her side throughout. It was nice to see a young couple super excited to introduce life to the world. That's where the pleasantness ends. Not for the loving couple, but for me. Some deliveries are clean and go smoothly. My first delivery was anything but. Trying to explain without being too graphic is difficult. Needless to say, every time she pushed, some stool would get expressed. I'm being a tad facetious, as to be more accurate the word "some" should be replaced with "a horse load." It had to have been a month since her last bowel movement. Each push, the pile at her feet grew and grew along with the stench. The nurse and I would continue to clean the pile and then replace our gloves with new ones over and over again. Eventually the baby's head started to show, and this literal shit show could come to an end. The attending gynecologist stood in the far corner never giving instruction. I had watched a lot of deliveries, but in reality I didn't know what the hell I was doing. The only thing I remembered was near the last push by the patient when the baby was nearly all the way out, I should actually apply some pressure and push the head slightly back in the vaginal opening as otherwise the baby could shoot out. What is actually more important is positioning your body up very close to the birth canal so a large gap isn't between you and the mother. This is important for two reasons. First, the doctor can use his hip or belly to help hold a very slippery baby. Secondly, you don't want a gap where the baby could fall through. Of course, I didn't remember this at the time. I was standing a bit too far back. I was trying to avoid the feces at my feet and not really wanting to get right up next to the vaginal orifice. The moment was upon us and she gave a final push. I gave slight pressure in the opposite direction and the baby slid right into my hands. Unfortunately, I did not use my arms or side of my body to aid stability. No, I was only using my slick hands extended from my body trying to hold this slimy, crying thing. Well, the greasy baby left my hands and all I could picture was the pile of excrement at my feet. "GET AHOLD OF THAT BABY, DOCTOR!" The gynecologist's first words in an hour. The baby continued to squirt out of my hands, but I was determined not to drop it. I would attempt to catch it every time it squirted free and after five steps and four near fumbles, I was standing in front of the new dad holding his bundle of joy. I had it secured, or so I thought. The dad didn't realize how close I had come to dropping it. I relaxed before handing the baby to the dad, a major mistake. Once again the baby started to slide out of my grip. "DOCTOR HOLD THAT BABY!" was shouted at me by the only actual doctor in the room. I was fumbling with the greasy thing and back stepped to where I had started. Right above the pile of poop. The baby fell through my hands completely, and dropped into the gynecologist's hands a few feet above a brown splash down. He pulled it into his hip and cradled it in his arms securely. "Nice hand off, Doctor. Let's give mom her new baby girl!" my attending said.

The happy couple didn't realize how close I came to dropping their baby, not once but multiple times. When I think about delivering a baby, a flood of bad memories hit me. They include mind numbing terror, associated with a foul stench permeating the entire area, and pure worry of dropping the little slime ball onto a pile of shit. The only fun thing I recall was what the new daddy told his girlfriend as she was holding her brand new baby girl, "Let's name her Jesse, after my favorite wrestler who an hour ago was voted the next governor of Minnesota."

5AM

I rush back to Room 8 to tell Big John he needs to save me from one of my biggest phobias. In this case, a delivery of a young woman who didn't have any prenatal care, is in complete denial, and whose father will most likely be killing the baby's daddy upon hearing the new revelation. I can kill two birds with one stone. I need to be present for the injecting of the sedation medicine for the hymenectomy to begin. I enter Room 8 and tell Judy to push the Versed. While the medicine is starting to take effect, I give Big John the details of my laboring denial patient. I think my voice isn't cracking much when I give him the story. Even with his hands full, he reassures me that he will check in shortly on my pregnant patient. I correct him and gently say, "You mean your new pregnant patient who will soon be leaving my ER!" I was giving him complete ownership of that one. I had no problem with helping deliver the avocado, but an actual baby, I wanted no part of.

The young girl with retained menses blood is soon no longer able to keep her eyelids open. She is set up in the stirrups and a surgical tray is arranged between her legs. The respiratory technician has her hooked up to oxygen delivered by nasal cannula, which is a plastic tube that ends in two prongs that stick into the base of her nostrils, where the oxygen is administered. Blood pressure, heart rate, and her oxygen saturations were continuously being monitored.

While I am in 8, Sharon knocks and enters. "Doc, an 18-year-old female with a swallowed foreign body checked in. She won't tell me what is stuck but said it's large, and she's acting embarrassed. I know you are busy and she looks fine waiting. Should I order soft tissue neck X-rays?"

I trust Sharon's judgment, and by the time I get free, the X-ray might be sitting at my desk to read, which would be excellent. "Sounds like a great idea, thanks Sharon," I answer. "Oh, let me know when the surgeon shows for my avocado guy," I add.

Sharon heads back out and quickly closes the door. Thankfully, Big John waited a minute for Sharon to leave. He was about to make his first incision and we did not want to put this unlucky girl on display. Hell, we also didn't want to expose any unfortunate passerby to a traumatic visual either. He makes a small hole in her hymen using a scalpel blade. I am bracing myself for the nastiest smell I have ever encountered. There is a good chance she had multiple months' worth of menstrual blood accumulating over time behind that tissue. I know all too well what odors spew forth after a one-month tampon has been exhumed. A trickle that quickly turned into a stream of dark brown fluid starts to drain into the basin placed on the ground below her groin. I am still awaiting the stench, but no odor followed. Incredibly, this old blood had no smell associated. It had been completely entrapped and was fluid that had never been exposed to any elements. It was the exact color of motor oil and I bite my tongue before I say something inappropriate. Reason being was, the patient's mom happens to be sitting by her daughter's side, holding her hand.

"I'll let things drain completely before I perform the full surgical procedure," Big John announced to all of us. "Adams, if you don't mind introducing me to the girl in labor. Oh, and Judy, come get me when the draining stops. Thanks."

Big John and I walk out of the room. I was still reveling in the fact that my olfactory senses were not bombarded with nausea-inducing badness. I escort Big John to Room 4 and we both enter. Melody looks a bit frazzled. I hope bringing the obstetrician with me will allow her to relax. I am so much more at ease now that Big John is at the bedside of the laboring patient. It is almost as if I took a tranquilizer. Next shift, when I call Big John to consult, I'll inform him of the analogy. He'll get a kick out of me telling him he was my giant Valium, calming my frantic nerves. I walk out after the introduction and can tell by the look in both daughter and mom's eyes they also feel more comfortable in Big John's presence. My anxiety must have been palpable.

I walk out of Room 4 and see my surgeon with his posse in Room 3's doorway. YES! A perfect trifecta to end the shift. Odor-free vaginal motor oil, baby delivery savior Big John, and now multiple surgical personnel to assist in avocado removal. I almost wanted to start dancing. I was definitely happy, but most likely the lack of sleep was making me a little punchy. "Adams, I brought my crew and chips. Are you making your famous guac?" the surgeon asks, laughing at his own joke. I smile because of my current jovial state, not his attempt at humor.

"It is deeper than my finger length," I tell all of them as I lift up my index finger. The surgeon's physician assistant's face is unreadable. The surgical resident looks excited, while the female medical student looks totally grossed out. "Once you are all set, I'll have Melody push some sedation and pain med. The respiratory tech is finishing a procedure with Big John next door in 4," I joyfully inform them. They get to go spelunking and I'll be solely responsible for sedation, or the new arriving ED doctor will.

As the five of us walk in, my patient with the anal foreign body gasps. "What! Did you tell everybody to come down and look at the freak?" he gripes.

I ignore his comment and get right down to business. "Dave, he sign the consent?" Dave nods a yes response. "Great, give him 5 mg Versed and put some oxygen on. Before we give another 5 mg, see if respiratory can step in," I state. I understand the patient is not happy, but removing the anal foreign body should make him content and people don't remember anything after getting a lot of Versed.

Sharon knocks and steps into the room. "Doc, um your X-ray on the swallowed foreign body is on display at your desk. Without GI on, you might want the surgeon to come take a look with you," Sharon informed us.

Back then we still used an X-ray illuminator or light box. I have not seen one used for many years. Now every ED has computer screens that bring up the scanned X-ray images. With computers, we can invert, magnify, and compare old images in seconds. The old school way used to be boxes on the wall that would light up when an X-ray film was slid into the slot and a back light would project through, allowing illumination of your recently taken film. Back then, if I had a question about something seen on the X-ray, I or a staff member would have to hand deliver the film to the radiologist so he could examine it. Today, multiple doctors can look at the same image on different continents minutes after the X-rays are taken. I walk back to my desk to look at the displayed X-ray image. The surgeon and his entourage are a few steps behind. I approach my desk and even before I am ten feet from the wall display, the foreign body is obvious. Seconds later I notice my ED tech Javier, Jan from radiology who took the X-ray, Cindy, Brandy, and a couple people I don't recognize, are also staring at the image. (X-ray image included, so you can see for yourself what we were all looking at.)

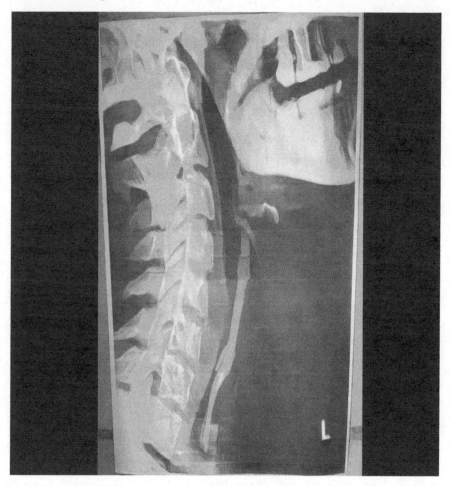

Yup, my new patient had swallowed a toothbrush and one that seems as dense as bone tissue. Plastic does not show up as visible as bone. This toothbrush must be laced with something as dense as bone, possibly metal? "Well, I'll go get the whole story and have Sharon start an IV. Good thing you brought your entire gang this morning," I say while addressing the surgeon. The surgical group joined the audience that was still staring at the X-ray image.

The surgeon takes it in stride by responding, "Well, it wouldn't be complete without the book end for our anal foreign body." Once again his PA is straight faced, the surgical resident is giddy, and the student is rethinking her career choice.

Sharon leads the way to Room 9 with me hot on her heels. We knock and enter together. I take a seat on the stool near the bed. Swallowed foreign bodies are very common, I would have to say a stuck fish bone is what I have had to remove the most often. An ingested coin is by far the most frequent, but they almost always pass without intervention. Worth mentioning is the dangerous button battery that on X-ray can mimic a coin. Those are time sensitive foreign bodies that if not removed may end a child's life. With the not-as-rare-as-you'd-think toothbrush FB, we have a little more time. They are used as a vomit aid by engaging the gag reflex, so will get swallowed from time to time.

The young woman looks slightly embarrassed, but is also smiling and in good spirits. Something tells me my new patient was using the toothbrush for something other than inducing vomiting. "Hi, I'm Dr. Adams. You seem to be tolerating that toothbrush in your esophagus pretty well."

She smiles, spits a tiny amount of saliva in the towel she is holding and then answers with, "I don't have much of a gag reflex and well, yesterday I bought the brand-new iPhone 3GS. It has video." She stops there as if that explained everything. I look at Sharon to see if she was as perplexed as I. Sharon's face looked like a combination of concern mixed with bewilderment. Sharon and I were not into new tech. We both had heard of the new smartphones and I had planned to purchase one soon, but they advanced so fast, I wasn't sure when I should jump in and buy one, or wait a while.

Unlike the phone technology, where I was hesitantly thinking of dipping my toe into a cold pool before jumping in, I decided to take the plunge by questioning my patient without beating around the bush. "What were you videotaping?"

She starts to giggle, then explains, "Well, because of what happened earlier tonight, I had some free time. So, I decided to make a video of myself, you know. Um, deep throating my toothbrush." She says it so matter-of-factly, I almost fall off my chair. Sharon starts laughing.

I have to plow straight ahead or I would be joining in the hysteria. "A toothbrush is not something that you will be able to poop out. So, Sharon is going to place an IV and give you medication. I already showed the surgeon your X-ray and he will take a tube with a camera on it down your throat and pull the toothbrush back out, ok?"

She looks over at Sharon, then back to me before she answers, "That sounds fine. I'm sorry I swallowed it and became such a bother."

This silly young girl was so sweet, I actually became envious of her boyfriend. Not for the reasons that you think either. "You will be getting sedation medicine and somebody will need to drive you home. Did someone drive you here?" I ask her.

She starts to answer, "My boyfriend's mom drove me because..."

Before she could complete her answer, Cindy knocked and shouted through the closed door, "Dr. Adams, Dr. Wang on Line 1 for you."

I stand up from the stool. "Excuse me, I have a phone call." I walk back to my desk. Why is Wang calling me? He should have finished the circumcision after the penis fracture case, hours ago. Because of those more urgent cases, I know the kid missed prom, but Wang should be home by now. I pick up the phone, "Hi Dick, what's up?"

"Hey, I have a message for you. I don't understand, but he is very adamant. My bling boy that I snip snip. Well, he had a little bleed last night in OR and so kept overnight and rechecked his hemoglobin. All good so he goes home now. I round early because golf tourney. Anyhow, I tell him he discharged and he said how long it take. I say may take an hour or so. He says his phone no work in hospital and he needs to get message to you."

I went from slightly confused to totally baffled. "Go on," I say.

Wang continues, "Well, his mom say girlfriend in your ED now. He tell me to tell you, don't throw away his toothbrush. It cost $300. You know what hell talking about?"

The mystery is solved. "I got it Dick, thanks. Tell the bling boy we won't throw it away. Oh, and have a great round of golf," I wish him luck before hanging up. Many things were answered with that phone call. The metal that lit up on the toothbrush X-ray I bet is gold. I also wager that she was showing off her skills that put him in the zipper predicament in the first place. My surgeon is going to love this story. He deserves to hear it all, since he will be the one doing the fishing.

5:50AM

I look up at the clock and am so happy I almost shed a tear. The EMS radio blares and my heart rate doesn't budge. They won't arrive on the scene until after 6AM, no reason to even listen. In addition, I have already decided I'm not touching my charts. I'll come in an hour early for the next shift. "Cindy, who is replacing me at 6?"

Cindy looks at the calendar schedule. "Looks like Dr. Lopez is on."

Awesome, she always arrives five minutes early each shift. I inform the surgeon's PA to save the toothbrush as I go check on Big John.

John is leaving his labor patient's room and looks a little concerned. He tells me, "Baby is breech and monitor shows some late decelerations, so I'm taking her up for a C-section. Everything should be fine, but I have to wait until 7AM for the new OR crew. You kept last night's crew too busy. Oh, can you give the pediatrician a heads up?" John smiles as he goes to finish the hymen patient's procedure. John turns around part way down the hall and says, "I'm still planning to golf, so tell your replacement only to call for real emergencies!"

I march back to my desk to call the pediatrician. Dr. Presley is the "kid or baby doctor" today and the favorite to win today's golf tourney. I get him on the phone and inform him of the 7 AM C-section, letting him know the patient was in pregnancy denial and had no prenatal care. He surprises me by revealing he sees a patient like this every year. I'm too tired to be shocked. I hang up the phone with one question on my mind. When is my replacement going to walk in? Seconds later the question is answered, as I see the new ER doctor at the door. There is nothing better than seeing your replacement arrive a few minutes before the end of a tough shift. I give Dr. Lopez a huge smile and start detailing what is left in the ED. I don't give her any time to even say hello.

"Am I glad to see you. Everyone left has a dispo. A lidocaine overdose patient should be leaving observation soon. I'll peek in on her before I leave. You only need to be aware, Big John has two patients and so does the surgeon. John is draining motor oil from a teenager in 8, she will go home within the hour. In Room 4, he will be taking a breech baby up for a 7AM C-section. I have notified the pediatrician. The surgeon and his posse are delivering an avocado in Room 3 and then will do an EGD (upper endoscopy) to fish for a pricey toothbrush in Room 9. You'll only have to provide sedation assistance for the surgeon's cases. Almost forgot! The father of the girl going for C-section doesn't know his daughter is pregnant. If he asks how she is, tell him she's doing fine and that he will be a grandpa by the time they start serving breakfast in the cafeteria. You may want to call the police to come in when you tell him, so he doesn't kill the new baby daddy.

Lopez's eyes bug out as she says, "So you had a crazy shift?"

I laugh and respond, "UNFORGETTABLE!"

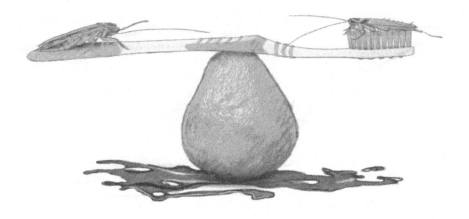

Epilogue

I enter my truck, sitting down while I place my stethoscope and lunch box on the passenger seat. I turn the ignition and flip the radio on. I am excited, knowing that Sunday morning at 6 AM they play 80s hits. Before I leave the hospital parking lot, Madonna's song, "Like a Virgin" starts playing. After my shift, the song seems to have new meaning for me. I almost turn it off, but realize I need to embrace the absurdity. I crank the volume and laugh. Reflecting back on the shift, I realize things could have been much worse. People don't go to the ER for a good time, but they do end up there when they have had too much of a "good time." So, if at the end of a shift everybody survives, and pain and suffering were alleviated, you can consider it a positive night's work. In addition, my staff was rock solid all night long. Of course, a few of the patients and visitors were also rock solid and in one case, not solid enough. What's more, with one unexpected baby on the way, more patients will be leaving the hospital than actually came through the ER doors. I would have to say it was a successful shift.

To you, the reader, I hope I was successful in my goal of providing entertainment with added education. Specifically, I was focused on adult readers with no medical background. I did, at times, write using more vernacular verbiage so the transition to medical terminology would not be so cumbersome. Also, you now have an idea of the employees who call the hospital's ED their workplace. Their primary job description is to bring aid to people when they are at their most scared, vulnerable, and suffering. My intention was not to make fun of or demean the patients I described, but to use their plights in hopes of providing medically educational insight, with

215

some of their racy entertaining examples of what can happen when genitals suffer injury, things get stuck, or when orgasms turn nasty.

After the drive home that early morning, I opened up the cabinet to grab a box of cereal. I usually eat a large bowl, and then minutes later my head hits the pillow. As I opened the fridge, I saw a can of beer next to the milk. I contemplated choosing the beer to pour on my cereal instead of the milk. That morning I didn't select the beer. Years later after an actual dreadful shift, I did substitute the beer for the milk, but that is a story for another time.

Abbreviations

ED	Emergency Department = ED
ER	Emergency Room = ED
PA	Physician Assistant
NP	Nurse Practitioner
CT/CAT	Computed Tomography
IV	Intravenous
CC	Chief Complaint
YO	Years Old
FB	Foreign Body
US	Ultrasound
OR	Operating Room
MG	Milligram
EMS	Emergency Medical Services
ET tube	Endotracheal Tube
LP	Lumbar Puncture
SAH	Subarachnoid Hemorrhage
CSF	Cerebrospinal Fluid
ECG/EKG	Electrocardiogram
STEMI	ST Elevation Myocardial Infarction
MI	Myocardial Infarction
BP	Blood Pressure
PVC	Premature Ventricular Complex
ICU	Intensive Care Unit
CK	Creatine Kinase
Rhabdo	Rhabdomyolysis
RN	Registered Nurse
LPN	Practical Nurse Degree
MDMA	Methamphetamine, Ecstasy/Molly
IM	Intramuscular

RA	Rheumatoid Arthritis
MS	Multiple Sclerosis
NS	Normal Saline
NPO	Nothing By Mouth
SCT	Sickle Cell Trait
LET	Lidocaine Epinephrine Tetracaine
EMLA	Lidocaine Prilocaine Anesthetic
TAC	Tetracaine Adrenalin Cocaine
CC	Milliliter
PID	Pelvic Inflammatory Disease
UTI	Urinary Tract Infection
hCG	Human Chorionic Gonadotropin
Rh	Rhesus factor (Blood Type)
IUP	Intrauterine Pregnancy
OB	Obstetrician
PAC	Premature Atrial Contraction
QRS	Main Spike on EKG (ventricle depolarization)
V-Tach	Ventricular Tachycardia
V-Fib	Ventricular Fibrillation
CPR	Cardiopulmonary Resuscitation
DNR	Do Not Resuscitate
UA	Urinalysis
MRSA	Methicillin Resistant Staph Aureus
E. coli	Escherichia Coli
CHF	Congestive Heart Failure
CTT	Cricothyroidotomy
CDC	U.S. Centers For Disease Control and Prevention
LGBTQ	Lesbian Gay Bisexual Transgender Queer
HPV	Human Papillomavirus
STD	Sexually Transmitted Disease

BPH	Benign Prostatic Hyperplasia
GI	Gastrointestinal
FHR	Fetal Heart Rate
BPM	Beats Per Minute
EGD	Upper Endoscopy

NOTES: